FABULOUS

Jelly

USE YOUR BRAIN
TO LOSE WEIGHT

SUSANNAH HEALY

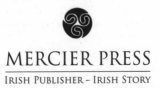

MERCIER PRESS
IRISH PUBLISHER – IRISH STORY

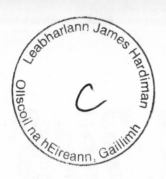

MERCIER PRESS

Cork

www.mercierpress.ie

© Susannah Healy, 2013

ISBN: 978 1 78117 180 6

10 9 8 7 6 5 4 3 2 1

Printed and bound in the EU.

FABULOUS
Jelly

For my parents, my siblings,
my husband and my children.

I love you endlessly.

CONTENTS

Introduction

I challenge you to find someone in Ireland who doesn't know roughly what constitutes a healthy diet and what we should be eating more or less of: less saturated fats, more fruit and veg., etc. So why is it that about forty per cent of the Irish population are still overweight? Well, possibly because all the diet and eating programmes doing the rounds require willpower, self-control and a healthy dollop of self-denial. But psychological research tells us that willpower is like money: spend it and it runs out. So what use is the endless expert advice about good nutrition if most of us simply can't manage to follow it? It seems that the gap between good nutrition and the reality of our daily lives is just too great. We all know what we're supposed to do, but never quite manage it. Or we choose to go 'all out' … starting next week, because we need time to guzzle every delicious food that we love but are going to give up forever when the diet starts.

Diet gurus talk about the need for a 'complete change of lifestyle' a 'lifestyle overhaul' and a 'new you'. This is an enormous ask of anyone and smacks of New Year's resolution speak – and we all know how long they last. Many of these eating programmes are drawn up by people who have no personal experience of the heart-breaking battle that a dieter goes through each time they start and then flunk a new diet. These programmes fail to acknowledge, and work with, the weaknesses in human nature, particularly in relation to all-out change.

As you read this book you will see that I am a great fan of Unislim, Weight Watchers and similar weight-loss clubs – they have done wonders for many people's lives. But most of their members will testify to how much easier it is to lose weight when we feel 'in the zone', i.e. that wonderful feeling of enthusiasm and motivation, when what you do and what you want seem to effortlessly line up together and your weight-loss goals are suddenly achievable. This book is about this piece of the puzzle: how to find the motivation to start losing weight. Based on my own personal experience and my professional insights as a psychologist, the Fabulous Jelly programme will help you to find the motivation to start losing weight NOW.

In case you have picked up this book simply

wondering what on earth 'Fabulous Jelly' is, I shall put you out of your misery. Fabulous Jelly refers to your brain; that phenomenal gelatinous lump that weighs around three and a half pounds, contains 100 billion neurons, 100,000 miles of blood vessels, is home to 100,000 chemical reactions every SECOND and an estimated one quadrillion separate pieces of information over a lifetime.[1] The brain is generally considered by scientists to be the most complex phenomenon in the universe – and you've got one. Unfortunately, most of us never even attempt to understand how it works; we treat it somewhat like the heating in a building, we know when it's on but that's about it. I hope that this book will help you to become aware of your amazing brain and how it affects your eating habits and weight-loss goals in particular.

I think you will find that the Fabulous Jelly programme is a breath of fresh air compared to what has gone before. It is based on my own experience of what worked for me and why, as well as really getting a leg up from the field of psychological research into why and when we eat. Please remember that I am not a dietician or nutritionist and to make the right food choices in the long term you may want to enlist the help of one of these professionals. Also, don't be naive about it. Eating *is* a matter of life and death so if you have any medical condition at all check with your doctor first before changing your diet.

A Bit About Me

I can't tell you how often I personally had a 'last supper' – the big 'last treat' before starting the diet the next day. I'm a chocoholic. There are plenty of things I like to eat, but chocolate is the clear winner. And I don't like anyone messing with my chocolate – I don't want it diluted with flour and eggs in a cake and I don't want it filled with wafer, toffee or any other substance that might take up space that could otherwise be filled by chocolate. So my 'last suppers' usually entailed a cup of tea and an enormous slab of chocolate broken off a giant bar picked up while queuing at the counter of some supermarket. When I was a child these huge bars, like the packets of sweets which hang on racks from the display unit, were called 'family packs', but somehow they now seem to have morphed into single servings. If the cup of tea wasn't available, the bar would sit in a cupboard or in the car so that I could nibble away at it continuously throughout the day. Of course, I often never quite managed to start the diet the next day – or I had started and stopped by lunchtime.

Many years ago I lost three stone with Weight Watchers. It was easy. I followed the system, got loads of exercise (which was also easy as I was a student at the time) and attended my meetings. From memory I don't think there was ever a week that I didn't lose weight and I could never quite understand how other people at the meetings found it so difficult. It seemed so simple to me: follow the plan and lose the weight. Fast forward ten years, I'm a busy working mother with neither the time nor the energy to stick to much of an eating or exercise plan. Somehow the motivation to eat healthily seemed to escape me. I was never a fan of set menu plans so instead I told myself that I would stop nibbling between meals or cut out carbs or never eat chocolate again or stop all sugary snacks completely. All good enough plans in moderation, but I never stuck to them. In fact, I never believed from the start that I would stick to them, so I often just told myself that this was being unkind to myself or unrealistic and jumped off the wagon and into a bar of chocolate. I joined and re-joined Weight Watchers countless times. I knew I had to devise a plan that 'knew me' – who I am, how I live my life and how I tick. I didn't want a whole 'new me'. In other matters not pertaining to eating I considered myself a fairly competent and together kind of person. I just wanted to lose weight.

If weight loss was a simple matter of 'eat less, exercise more' we would all need only one diet book. We all know it should be simple maths: calories in, calories out. But it isn't. In order to start moving more and eating less we need to get in 'the zone', in the mood or simply disgusted enough with ourselves to finally shift ourselves into gear. This book is about that bit. Weight loss isn't a 'journey'. Travelling to France is a journey. So is watching countries go by while sitting in the dining car of the Trans-Siberian railway. Weight loss can feel more like an Iron Man Decathlon – this book is about getting up off the couch and into the runners. The distance you choose to go is up to you. I was inspired to write this book by all the times I thought about losing weight, yet did nothing, and by the technique I finally found of jumping into 'the zone' and keeping myself motivated enough to keep going – surprisingly with great ease. As I said, in the rest of my life I tick along just fine. So the fact that week after week, month after month, and particularly, Monday after Monday I would consider, contemplate and then ditch the idea of starting to lose weight really irritated me. Why was it so hard to lose weight? Of course, I knew (and you, the reader know) the risk of lots of nasty diseases associated with excess weight and I waited for the day when my own bottom would feature on one of those documentaries on obesity that film the backs of lots of faceless pedestrians walking down some street. (And everyone has that 'friend' who will be sure to tell you that your bottom was on the telly!)

I'm not a dietician or a nutritionist so you may well want to contact one of these. I didn't write this book to repeat all the stuff you already know about what you should and shouldn't eat. If you don't know it by now there are plenty of books out there to help you with that bit. This book is written for the millions of people who already know all of that but just can't quite get it together to get started. I was one of you.

This book tells you how I finally started to work out what was and wasn't going on in my head that was keeping me out of 'the zone': that gorgeous feeling when suddenly weight loss seemed easy and I wondered why I hadn't started ages ago. To get to this point you will need to delve into your thoughts to find out what is preventing you from making the changes you need to make. Luckily you can do this in private, keeping the messy bits to yourself. I want to show you that all the corset-wearing, army-drilling, boot-camping (now there's an interesting picture!) in the world won't help you to achieve your desired healthy weight unless you have sought permission from the 'control tower' – your brain.

Using some basic concepts of psychological therapy, such as cognitive behavioural therapy and other areas of psychological research, I will help you to develop an eating plan that works with, not against, your unconscious instincts, needs, habits and motivations, so that your mind will allow you to gently change the habits of a lifetime.

Please be sensible about how you put the recommendations of this book into practice. Of course, if you are morbidly obese, a diabetic or suffer from any other medical condition, you should refer to your medical practitioner before changing your diet.

In fact, I am not prescriptive about what you can eat – you can largely choose according to your own personal preferences. What I do here is give some insight into why other eating plans haven't worked for you and what things you need to include in any eating plan you choose in order to make it work. Albert Einstein once defined insanity as doing the same thing over and over again and expecting different results. The same applies to weight loss. There's no point embarking on yet another diet if you're going to use the same mental apparatus. This book will help you gain an insight into what you need to change. In addition, the eating plan outlined here is not a life-long eating plan: go to a properly qualified dietician for that. The Fabulous Jelly programme aims to help you to see fast results without denying yourself the things you really love. Once you have lost the initial weight you have something worth protecting and you'll suddenly realise that that bag of crisps, mountain of pasta or Chinese take-away just isn't worth losing your new figure for. That's when your life-long eating habits will change – effortlessly.

The Fabulous Jelly programme does not aim to get you a perfectly toned beach-ready body, but it will get you back within a healthy weight range for your height and age (BMI).

However, you do not need to read all of *Fabulous Jelly* if you feel like starting to eat differently today. Just do it! Grab your motivation and let it take you where you want to go, starting right now. The rest of us will be plodding somewhere behind you until we feel our own motivation sweep us off our feet – but we will see you at the finish line.

1

gNATs in Your Head

We all have them. Invisible, sneaky, forever reproducing and hard to catch, these little bug***s cause a lot of problems. (gigantic) Negative Automatic Thoughts (gNATs) are habits in our thinking that we are not even aware of. Picked up from parents, people we are close to and life experiences, these negative ways of thinking can become so automatic (unconscious) to us that we rarely get a chance to challenge them. They colour how we view our lives, others, situations, ourselves – and food. Think about how many assessments you make about things every day that guide how you live. For example you might say to yourself:

It would be just my luck if the bus was on time today when I'm running late.

Or

What if that other guy going for interview has a better CV than me?

Or

I'm always coming out with the wrong thing or putting my foot in it.

Or

I'm bound to be the one that doesn't meet anyone special.

Most people never learn that how they think is, in fact, just one way of seeing things and that if our thoughts aren't working for us we can learn to choose an alternative way of thinking. This is great news! Imagine dumping all the huge, years-out-of-date generalisations that you make about yourself and the world, and replacing them with kinder and more accurate statements that relate to you on one particular day in one particular situation.

For example, 'I'm rubbish at public speaking' becomes 'I had one, or a few, bad experiences at public speaking when I was really nervous because I had no training/wasn't prepared, but I presume that if I got training I'd be just as good as others who have more experience than me.'

Of course, dumping out-dated or inaccurate statements about yourself can work in the opposite direction, e.g. just because your adoring mother said you should wear your hair in a high ponytail doesn't mean that you still should twenty years later. Similarly you may have had to 'put meat on your bones' when you were a scrawny seven-year-old boy, but perhaps any more meat on your bones now and you could be a one-man threat to the environment.

Two of the most important ideas in cognitive behavioural therapy are:

THOUGHTS ARE NOT FACTS

and

YOU FEEL THE WAY YOU THINK

so ...

IF YOU DON'T LIKE HOW YOU'RE FEELING

(E.G. BEACHED WHALESQUE)

... CHANGE HOW YOU ARE THINKING!

The biggest gNATs when it comes to overeating are:

1. Over-Generalising: Do you catch yourself saying things like: *'I'm big. It's just the way I'm made. We're all like this in my family …'*?

Oh really? So your eating habits have nothing to do with your size? Do you actually eat very healthily? Do you get plenty of exercise? Do you eat similarly to the rest of your family? Do you eat 'treat' foods given to you as a child? Do your siblings? Do you run around as much as you did when you were a kid? Do you have the same metabolism as you did when you were young? Of course you don't. And having a round-shaped face is NOT the same as being chubby-faced or a spare chin collector. The chances are if you and your siblings are all overweight you probably all learned the same poor eating habits and attitudes to food and exercise. You're not made that way, you just learned it that way. Your ideas about eating aren't fact, they are opinions – and they're not working for you so it's time for a change. (If you sincerely believe that you might have a medical problem that contributes to your weight gain, then obviously you need to discuss this with your doctor.)

OR

'I hate exercise …'?

All exercise? Do you hate walking on the seafront on a sunny afternoon? Do you hate walking around your local park while catching up on the gossip with a pal? What games did you play outside with friends as a child? Do you support any sports teams? Chances are you don't hate all exercise, you just either haven't tried enough different types of exercise to find the one for you or you simply hate the feeling of being out of breath that you get now when exerting yourself. That bit is understandable. But don't expand it out to hating exercise in general. Saying you dislike the shortness of breath you feel while running too fast now that you are unfit/overweight is a more accurate statement. It also instantly sounds like something more temporary and gets you thinking about ways you could get over the problem, like starting with walking, or jogging so slowly to begin with that you're barely moving forward with each step, or walking with a friend so you are distracted by the chat, or getting coaching in a sport you have an interest in so that there's loads of stopping and starting and plenty of time to catch your breath. All of these options offer you a way out of the habit of thinking in generalisations.

2. Fortune Telling – Predicting the Future: Do you tell yourself things like: *'I'm just bound to put the weight back on. I always do ...'*?

Think about the times this happened before. Exactly how many times have you lost weight then put it back on again? What did the diet(s) involve? What were the main changes you had to make to your previous eating habits? Did the programme involve 'all-or-nothing' thinking? Did it involve extremes, i.e. 'completely cut out x'? Did it fit in with your average day or did it require a lot of changes and self-discipline? Did it wreck your weekends? So many eating plans seem to think that a person can make a full-time job of their weight-loss plans, so don't blame yourself if it didn't work for you. We all know what we should and shouldn't be eating so if those previous diets you tried just regurgitated all the same information you could have got from the Internet then don't just presume that no eating plan will ever work for you. What did you learn from your previous attempts at weight loss? Which type of diet did you prefer – a set menu programme or something that allowed you more choice? What bits did you struggle with most? Did you feel hungry on some? How did you feel about that? Many people never leave long enough between meals to feel hungry and find the experience of eating when hungry really refreshing. Others just find they eat too much when hungry. Did any or all of your previous diets demand that you tried out new recipes? Did you enjoy trying new foods or do you now have a cupboard full of spices you can't pronounce and a mortgage-worth of rotten but rather exotic-sounding vegetables in your kitchen? Think about what you have learned from these experiences regarding what works for your lifestyle.

REMEMBER: YOU WILL START TO LOSE WEIGHT FOR GOOD WHEN YOU FIND A PROGRAMME THAT WORKS WITH YOUR LIFE INSTEAD OF ASKING YOU TO CHANGE YOUR LIFE.

3. Mental Filtering: Do you protect your current beliefs as if you were Flash Gordon defending the universe?

Mental filtering relates to our mind's dislike for change, which causes us to unconsciously think in a biased way. This means that we tend to take in only information that holds with our current beliefs and to dismiss information contrary to our current views, which results in us never updating our views of the world and ourselves.

Think about what mental filters you might be carrying with you through life without being aware of it. What are your beliefs relating to eating? (This is actually a really interesting exercise to do regarding all aspects of your life, but let's stick to eating for the moment.) Maybe you believe you have no self-discipline. If you hold this belief then you probably feel that you haven't a hope of succeeding on any weight-loss plan. You need to begin looking for information that contradicts this belief. For example, do you get out of bed each day? Do you produce a dinner for yourself and/or others each evening when you would rather spend the time in front of the TV? Do you get yourself to work/college every day?

'Ah, but I mean I have no self-discipline when it comes to denying myself my favourite foods,' I hear you say. So let's look at this more specific belief. Have you *ever* said no to another helping or decided to save that bar of chocolate until later in the day? Have you *ever* not stopped at a particular shop because you knew you would buy yourself something you shouldn't? Have you *ever* gone for a walk to get exercise? Have you *ever* gone easy on the carbs the day before a date so that you feel your best on the big night? Are you better at 'being good' earlier in the day but find your self-discipline fades later in the day? If you answer 'yes' to any of these questions then you do indeed have self-discipline, but you need to learn to identify when and where you can act with some discipline in your average day or week and where you fall down. You also need to update your information: most people's self-discipline fades when they get tired, or when they are placing other demands on themselves which also require self-discipline. So maybe previous eating plans didn't work for you because the programme demanded huge self-discipline and completely ignored the realities of human nature – most people's nature – not just yours.

STOP BEING SO HARD ON YOURSELF. THE CHANCES OF YOU BEING DIFFERENT TO EVERY OTHER HUMAN BEING ARE ZIP, SO IF OTHER PEOPLE CAN LOSE WEIGHT FOR GOOD, SO CAN YOU.

(We will be dealing with the subject of willpower in more detail in Chapter 8.)

We take on these statements about ourselves often without ever scrutinising them first. What's more, these beliefs become the markers by which all other new information about ourselves is judged. It's a bit like a giant filter or sieve we surround ourselves with which is quick to let in any information that's in keeping with our existing beliefs but slow to accept anything that contradicts them.

So, for example, if you think you can't sing and then on a Karaoke night out someone says you have a nice voice, you will dismiss the compliment as them just being polite. It would take several people complimenting you, probably on a number of different occasions, for you to begin to challenge your deeply held belief that you can't sing. However, a single throwaway joke from someone about your failings in the singing department will be fully taken on board because it's in keeping with your existing belief.

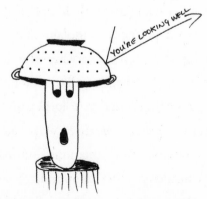

NIGEL'S MENTAL FILTER MEANT HE NEVER BELIEVED ANYONE WHO TOLD HIM HE WAS LOOKING WELL

4. Disqualifying the Positive: Do you have a tendency to forget about previous successes or negate them as unimportant or just luck?

This habit is related to mental filtering. For example, you may have lost weight before but then put some or all of the weight back on. Instead of seeing this as proof that you are able to lose weight you instead look upon the experience as a personal failure. Or perhaps you think that someone telling you how well you look is just them being polite. Or perhaps you are reading this in wintertime and telling yourself that it's the worst time of year to try to get some exercise outdoors instead of admitting that it's the very best time to start getting out there without bringing attention to yourself – think cap on/hood up, dark evenings – anonymity guaranteed! Be honest, if it were summer-time you'd probably complain that you hate going walking and seeing everyone else in skimpy little running gear and feeling like a blob as they lap you yet again going round your local park.

Start to become aware of what you say to yourself and how you view situations and experiences. You may consider yourself an optimist, but even optimists have their personal weaknesses, and negative self-beliefs about weight loss may well be yours.

5. All-or-Nothing Thinking: Do you think in extremes?

This is the *really* big offender when it comes to weight loss. All-or-nothing thinking involves thinking in extremes: seeing things as black or white while ignoring the multiple shades in between. Maybe you're either on a diet or else eating everything that stays still long enough for you to shovel it into your mouth. No gradual changes for you. Or maybe you decide that you won't start eating better until next week because you are going out on Saturday night so that wipes out the rest of this week as a consideration. Maybe you tell yourself you are 'being good today' or 'being bad today' in relation to your eating and take an 'I've started (the day eating rubbish) so I'll finish (the day the same way)' sort of approach to classifying the days of the week. Perhaps you think you won't feel good about yourself until you have lost a certain amount of weight, or use a perfectionist approach against yourself and refuse to go for a walk because you feel disgusted with yourself that you get out of breath.

TAKE THAT GIRDLE OFF YOUR BRAIN! QUIT THINKING IN SUCH RIGID TERMS AND GET SOME FLEXIBILITY BACK INTO YOUR HEAD.

Sometimes it is easier to be clear about the mental chit-chat going through your head by writing it down. You will probably find that when you commit this week/month/years/life-long self-talk to pen and paper it is the same few sentences being repeated again and again and again. These sentences often include the pros and cons of losing weight separated by a big 'BUT' in the middle. For example, someone might write:

'I want to lose weight BUT I couldn't give up having a few drinks at the weekend.'

Or

'I can lose weight Monday to Friday BUT I always put it back on at the weekend.'

Or

'I do want to lose weight BUT I honestly do not have the time for the exercise that everyone says is needed.'

Or

'I have no interest in losing weight BUT my

partner has clearly lost interest in me sexually and I'm scared of losing her/him.'

It is really important that all parts of these goals and concerns are considered valid and important. The beliefs and worries that come after the 'BUT' are just as important to you at the moment as the desire to lose weight stated at the start of the sentence. If they weren't they wouldn't hold you back from your goal. So now you need to write each of your self-talk statements again, replacing 'BUT' with 'AND'. This validates the concerns that are holding you back, brings them to the foreground and gives you the opportunity to address them. Now you have the starting point of a process of brainstorming and negotiation where you can look for all the shades of grey between your original black and white, all-or-nothing thinking.[2] We will be looking at ways to do this in later chapters.

6. Catastrophising: Do you make every setback an absolute catastrophe?

Do you give up trying just because you couldn't resist the obligatory side order of chips that come with every order of food in Ireland? Do you decide that there is no point looking after how you eat for the rest

33

of the week because of the kids' birthday party you were at yesterday where you ignored all the nibbles laid out for the adults and tucked into the sausages and chips, jellies, chocolate cake and ice cream meant for the kids? Do you look upon your twisted ankle that means you can't go walking as a reason for giving up on weight loss?

Shake off the extreme thinking. If you have chosen the right eating plan for you then you won't feel so under pressure to see results every week, because you won't be making huge sacrifices or changes to your lifestyle. Or maybe you will decide to take it easier on the fatty foods for the rest of the week. In fact, the more of these events you have, the more opportunities you have to learn to fit them into your eating plan rather than having to make your lifestyle fit with the eating plan.

'WOULD YOU LIKE CHIPS WITH YOUR CHIPS SIR?'

Like most people I love chips, but sometimes they just make my meal feel grotty. On one particular evening my husband and I ordered a family meal in a pub and asked specifically for no chips with our meals, knowing that we could always steal a few off the kids' plates if needed. Somehow the message didn't get back to the kitchen and both our meals arrived to the table with chips on the side. A few minutes later the waitress came back with an extra plate of chips 'just to keep everyone happy'. Six people and seven portions of chips! Of course we made a good dent in them before gathering the strength to ask for them to be taken away. But I still lost weight that week.

Beware of the very Irish epidemic of chips!

7. Mind Reading: Do you think you know exactly what other people will think or say about your weight-loss goals?

Do you stop making changes because you just know they'll be thinking 'here s/he goes again – another failed diet'? Do you believe you know that friends and/ or family presume you will fail? Do you avoid taking exercise because you think people passing in cars or others in the gym are commenting on your size?

GET OVER YOURSELF! You are not the centre of other people's universe. Because we are so important to ourselves we tend to presume that other people pay as much attention to us as we do. This is not the case. People you meet are mostly interested in themselves – not in a bad, selfish way – it's just a survival thing. So even the people close to you who ask about your new eating habits may either only be asking because they feel they have to show an interest, or may be interested but actually more interested in whether or not their favourite TV programme recorded successfully! The people who pass you in cars or on the bus may, or may not, register that you are there, but any thoughts of you will be quickly replaced by things of far more interest – like wondering if they drove a bit faster would that spider fall off their side mirror, or trying to decipher the obscenity graffitied on the bus seat in front of them. Sorry, but your weight-loss and exercise efforts are simply not that important to anyone else. Accept and enjoy friendly support when it is offered, but remember that you will probably not be in their minds twenty seconds later. Do not let your IMAGINED ideas about what others are thinking about you get in your way.

TAKING MYSELF OUT OF THE CENTRE OF THE UNIVERSE

It's amazing how we all fancy ourselves as the centre of everyone else's universe. I got married on a beautiful summer day and, as can be expected, I remember the day as being perfect, not just for me, but for everyone who was there. Others don't remember it quite that way.

One of my bridesmaids was pregnant at the time and often experienced sudden drops in blood sugar. She had got somewhat used to this and came prepared with some slim bars of chocolate packed tightly into the lining of her dress. She managed to get through the ceremony but on the drive back to the venue she knew she was in trouble and needed the chocolate fast.

Her most vivid memory of my wedding is of whipping the chocolate out of her dress and demolishing it while a stunned six-year-old flower girl looked on. She could stare all she wanted – she wasn't getting any. To this day I'm still not quite sure what would have happened had she needed the chocolate while at the altar!

Lesson learned:

We are not the centre of everyone else's universe

AND

Be Prepared!

gNATS are sneaky because they are unconscious. Now that you have read through the list you may find that you do them all, but most of us do at least some of them some of the time. Becoming aware of these habits in thinking, i.e. making them conscious, is the first step towards challenging them. But don't just have a quick read through this chapter and then carry on to the next. Take out pen and paper and write down a few things you say to yourself about losing weight and see if they could be labelled as gNATs. Sometimes a single statement may contain two or more types of gNATs. Label it, then challenge it. Look for evidence that contradicts it – even some of the time. Practise noticing how you talk to yourself every day and identify when you are using a gNAT. You should be feeling a lot more positive about your goals by the end of the exercise as well as feeling a bit chuffed about your newly acquired mind bending techniques that you can apply to other areas of your life.

And there you have it – all your excuses for failure and sitting on your behind doing nothing blasted out of the water!

2

MIND HOW YOU GO

(AND BEWARE OF THE CUTE HEURISTIC)

Did your mother ever tell you to be careful of dark shortcuts where it's difficult to see where you are going? Turns out she was probably more right than she knew.

Every day we are faced with countless decisions and assessments, some important and others trivial. For example, by the time you read this page today you will probably have decided whether or not you would hit the snooze button for the third time, what to wear, what to have for breakfast, which spoon to take out of the drawer, whether to listen to the radio or not, etc. You may also have made some bigger decisions like handing in your notice at work, or ditching your bank, supplier or other half. In order to cope with the onslaught of demand on your thinking capacity and preserve energy, your brain takes a few mental short-cuts by making many of these decisions using what are known as cognitive (thinking) heuristics.

Cognitive heuristics are general rules of thumb that your brain uses to simplify decision-making so that it doesn't have to work too hard reinventing the wheel as it were. Since you were a little new-born bundle of joy, your brain has been becoming the best pattern-matching machine the world has ever seen. From your earliest moments you had a template for what a human face should look like and were able to 'pattern-match' all the cooing globular shapes that peered into your cot to a 'what a human face looks like' template and were soon able to recognise them as people. If you had too specific a template for facial recognition you would not have been able to differentiate between different relatives. If you did not have such a template at all you might have confused those cooing faces with one of the many soft rattling round things that lay in your cot and tried to suck on someone's nose with unwanted, although also educational, results.

Pattern-matching also helps us in times of danger. Through personal experience, stories recounted by others and the media, we have learned (and some-times mis-learned) a number of cues for danger, such as darkness, being alone, raised and angry voices, etc. Due to our instinct for self-preservation, our brains are quick to learn about any potential dangers to us and particularly remember any memory with a strong emotion attached. (This is why your memories of your school days for example are likely to be made up of events with strong emotions, such as the time that guy in fifth year pulled up your skirt in full view of 400 other students, or the time your third class teacher made you stand up and read your poem to the school assembly, and so on.) If you are out walking at night and suddenly you notice that no cars are passing and you suddenly feel scared even though you have never had a bad experience before, your brain is pattern-matching signals for danger that you may have seen on television with your environment.

Unconscious pattern-matching also occurs in phobias. Sometimes a person develops a phobia of something that never used to cause them problems or feels anxious in situations for no apparent reason. *Sometimes* (and please don't apply this to every person's phobia or anxiety) this can be due to an unconscious cue in the environment that was present at another time when they really were in danger. For example, if a person is mugged while walking down a particular street then no one will be surprised if they don't feel much like walking down that street for some time afterwards. But sometimes they later feel panic in places that seem unrelated to their misfortune. What may be happening is that the unconscious mind will have taken in far more information about the mugging than the person remembers and is now pattern-matching something in the new environment to something it saw, felt or heard during the mugging. It may be as simple as a house with a green door or a cat that was on the street at the time. The person then experiences feelings of panic in a completely different place when they see a green front door or a cat sitting innocently on a garden wall.

When faced with imminent danger, our brain's ability to see a similarity (pattern) with previous knowledge about dangerous situations and get us the hell out of there without any conscious thought on our part is brilliant. That's one of the 'fabulous' bits. But, the ability to short-circuit the 'Will I run like hell? … no maybe I'm just imagining things … but I definitely heard a creepy noise … no, I'll just turn up my music a bit louder' dilly-dallying also results in a tendency to not bother looking at all the information when sizing up more everyday challenges. Instead our brain makes some bottom-rounding lazy decisions: like going for second helpings or avoiding running around the block again.

Patterns in how we think become our mental habits; if we see a similarity to a previous event or situation our brains will be only too delighted to turn on the autopilot and think as we always have. This means that unless we learn to recognise these biases in our thinking we can spend our entire lives functioning on a sort of autopilot mode. But like the gNATS, if we can learn to recognise when certain biases are creeping in then we can learn to involve the (hopefully) more logical, less instinctive part of the brain. Results may vary.

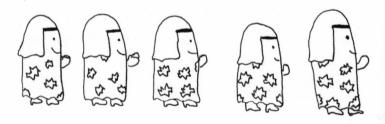

THE NEW HABIT PATTERN CAUGHT ON
QUICKLY IN THE CONVENT

Here are a few of the thinking habits relevant to eating that might ring a bell with you:

1. Unit Bias

How many times have you said that you're having 'a good day' or a 'bad day' when it comes to eating? This is the sort of Mastermind logic where you decide that 'I've started so I'll finish' (the day eating as much or as little as you first began). You look at the day as a unit so that if you began the day badly by eating more than you perhaps should have, you then decide that you will just keep going and start afresh tomorrow. Or worst of all you look at the entire week as a single unit so that if you don't quite manage the super-healthy breakfast you had planned on Monday morning you decide that this wasn't the week for you and you'll try again next week.

Feeling the need to clear your plate is another example of thinking of the dinner plate as one unit. Weight Watchers and other manufacturers have cottoned on to this tendency and now make boxes of biscuits with two biscuit portions individually wrapped inside. However, this tactic is no match for the determination of many, who move their view of the unit to the entire box.

CLIMBING UP THAT HILL

Unit bias can apply to anything and everything. When I finally started to build up the stamina to shuffle around my local park twice, I set my sights on managing a third lap. Unfortunately the direction I normally ran in began with a steep hill (OK, a slight incline) and for weeks I just couldn't get the energy together for the third lap. That third lap had become a 'unit' in my head without my realising it. I was either going to do it or not try at all. For ages it didn't occur to me to try a bit of it, to walk the hill and then return to my shuffle, to reverse my direction so that I could end the third lap on a downhill or any, now completely obvious, alternative. I had become utterly rigid in my thinking even though logically I should have known that I did have the energy reserves for the task as I normally also shuffled home from the park and could have chosen to 'spend' that energy on the third lap instead until I got used to it. It wasn't until I started to think about all the other ways I used unit-biased thinking that I recognised what I was doing in the park and was able to give myself some options. But I still hate that hill: two and a half minutes of pain!

2. Gut Instinct

Technically speaking it is called the 'affect heuristic' when we use our instant emotional response, such as fear, happiness, pleasure, etc., to guide our decision making; but it's better known as gut instinct. In some instances trusting our gut can be useful as we can unconsciously pick up on danger signals in our environment that we are not consciously aware of. But we are creatures of habit and some of those gut instincts are just demonstrations of our mind dragging its knuckles towards change, increased risk or effort, or any temporary decrease in things that bring us pleasure. Were your body a finely tuned instrument, I might suggest that you feel free to follow your gut instinct, but you would probably be too busy pounding the pavements, meditating or running for office to be reading this book anyway. No, sadly, were we to take a look at your visceral Oracle of Wisdom we are more likely to find a bubbling, frothy quagmire, which may indeed be home to some strange strains of life but whose opinions you might be less likely to follow were you somehow able to come face-to-face with them. Sometimes your gut is the laziest part of you – completely ignore it when it tells you to keep stuffing your face.

47

3. The Denomination Effect

This refers to our tendency to spend more money when it is denominated in small amounts rather than notes; however, it can also affect how we 'spend' our daily calories. When we sit down to a large meal we are more likely to pay attention to what we are putting in our mouths and make some sort of a mental deduction from the daily tot up. But if we prefer to graze through the day it becomes very easy to forget about some of the things we ate during the day as they, in and of themselves, may have been of small calorific value. But they add up. Many people are particularly prone to this with liquid calories, which somehow they don't seem to count when it comes to food intake. Juices, lattes, cappuccinos and fizzy drinks all contain sugar and can break the bank when it comes to weight loss. The same goes for all those mini-break type foods, like dips and especially diet yogurts that we often eat standing up at the fridge door. One a day might be OK (although remember when they take out fat they usually pour in more sugar), but just because one seems fairly innocuous doesn't mean that three or four of them won't add up. As in any budget, you need to watch the sneaky little things that seem to cost nearly nothing – they are the snakes in the grass of weight control.

4. The Effort Heuristic

Related to the denomination effect is the effort heuristic, which affects how we value things based on the amount of effort that we think went in to its making. For example, if you found €100 you might choose to blow it on a whim on the basis of 'easy come, easy go' type thinking. However, if you had to go to work for five hours to earn that €100 you are likely to be a lot more careful about how you spend it. The same applies to the daily food 'allowance' that you set yourself. Have you ever sweated and toiled on a treadmill in a gym only to see that you have actually burned fewer calories than are in a single biscuit? It's enough to make a rock cry, but it is a useful (albeit not very exact) exercise in terms of making us aware of the effort required to burn off that next latte, scone or tikka masala.

As one woman put it, 'It's not that I don't eat chips anymore. It's just that if the chips are cold I'll insist on getting a fresh hot portion. I no longer just eat everything because it's there or because I'm not "being good". I'm more discerning. I insist on making everything I eat enjoyable … making it count.'

THINK TWICE BEFORE YOU PUT IT IN YOUR MOUTH! IT ISN'T ROCKET SCIENCE. SPEND YOUR 'BUDGET' WISELY AND BE AWARE OF JUST HOW MUCH WORK YOU WILL NEED TO DO TO WORK IT OFF. THE REALITY IS YOU PROBABLY WON'T WORK IT OFF.

5. The Picture Superiority Effect

Are you still with me? Or are you still picturing that plate of chips? If the latter, then you may be succumbing to what is known as the picture superiority effect, which says that anything we see or imagine as a picture is far more likely to be remembered than words. Professional athletes take advantage of this principle all the time when they visualise carrying out their perfect shot, kick, hit, throw, etc. Our mind thinks in pictures.

For example: Close your eyes for ten seconds and don't think of a pink elephant.

What did you do? You probably instantly pictured a pink elephant and then perhaps tried to turn him to a different colour or into a different animal.

Why did this happen? Because the words 'pink elephant' have a picture linked to them but the word 'don't' doesn't. Your mind therefore jumped to the picture and then tried to correct itself. Add in a few more senses and you've created the most memorable and dangerous craving you could ever imagine. We'll talk more about cravings later, but in the meantime, as soon as you become aware that you are craving for something, change the visual to seeing a more negative image, such as the guilt or bloated feeling you get as you place the empty packet in the bin. Add in that 'Oh hell, I did it again' sense of kicking yourself for good measure. Or choose a more positive alternative, like thinking of yourself leaving that room in a few seconds time feeling delighted with yourself for protecting your weight loss achieved to date. Then stick an apple in your mouth if required and get out of there. We will talk about how mindfulness can help in a later chapter but, going back to a basic assumption of cognitive behavioural therapy, remember:

YOUR THOUGHTS ARE NOT FACTS

Look upon cravings as being separate from you. Like passing ships, they can be very attractive, but that doesn't mean you have to jump on board. Each thought or craving will pass and it would be preferable if you were not half a pound heavier when it does.

6. The Framing Effect

How we see things has a lot to do with the environment we are in at the time – this is what is known as the framing effect. For example, many of us would be tempted to see a plate of food with a salad and vegetables on the side as a healthy, balanced meal. Our eyes take a quick snapshot of the plate, we make an assumption and without much mental effort we label it as being healthy without taking the fat and sugar content of the rest of the meal into account. Or what about the bliss of Internet shopping that means we can completely avoid seeing ourselves in public dressing rooms and comparing ourselves to other-sized bodies; or going to plus-size clothing shops and choosing the smaller-sized clothes because in some cases it's better to be the small fish in the big pool? Do you have a scone every time you have a coffee with friends even though you would never have one when alone? Do you consider a dinner party or meal out a licence to pig out on stuff that you would never eat the rest of the week? These are all examples of times when your environment (the 'frame') affects how you see things, or you changed the environment to make it feel better to you – crafty, but not helpful.

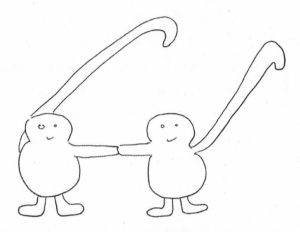

Do you view the world through the lens of your fat goggles?

Of course, some of the images we see through our fat goggles are just stereotypes – that well-known mental shortcut that clumps lots of people or things in together just because they have one thing in common. Some of these stereotypes might either be stopping you from changing your eating habits and getting up off the couch or else making the desired end result seem completely unachievable.

If your heart sinks at the very word 'diet' you probably have a number of negative assumptions about diets as being about deprivation, self-denial, hunger, etc. Take off the fat goggles and you might be able see the word 'diet' as describing what you eat in general – good, bad and indifferent. Perhaps you describe slim people as 'skinny minnys', as if being super skinny and being a healthy weight are the same thing. If you think that the end result of making a few changes to your eating habits is to turn yourself into your image of a skinny minny then you may just decide that you haven't a hope and won't bother trying. If this is the case try seeing yourself as still a little curvy but less than you are now – it's an easier sell to your unconscious (remember it is in charge and it will have the last say on the result). If you think that everyone who takes exercise is slim, walking or jogging fast and decked out in the most unforgiving shiny lycra, then you're not likely to chance leaving the house anytime before sundown. Next time you are out and about make a point of looking for people who don't fit that stereotype – the ones who look like they could do with a lift the rest of the way home. Phrases like 'I'm just not a runner' or 'it's just not me to join a club' are a sure sign of stereotyping. There is no runner/fitness/healthy eater 'type'. Put them all in a room for a day and they would probably kill each other. You are no different in being different to everyone else. Did I mention before that you need to get over yourself?

3

NO STRANGERS TO FAILUREVILLE

As I've mentioned, weight loss is usually a bit of an endurance challenge. Bring the subject up in conversation and you're likely to be talking and comparing diet plans and sympathetically listening to stories of each other's failures for the remainder of the day. In fact, it can be quite the social bonding exercise, but more on that later. The only other similar life event that comes close is giving up smoking, but as you can't give up eating completely, weight loss might seem like it wins hands down in the difficulty stakes. How mean would someone have to be to wave cigarettes in the face of someone who has recently given up saying, 'Go on, have one, you know you want to ...'? It just doesn't happen. But the equivalent happens every day for the dieter because they have to eat. Herein lies the good news: smokers have to give up cigarettes completely but YOU ARE NOT GIVING UP EATING! You are going to be able to dive wholeheartedly into gorgeous, delicious, warm, tasty meals every day for the rest of your life!

Sounds better?

But why do we all forget this?

There are two reasons:

1   Because we tend to have a visual image of healthy food as meaning hedges of lettuce and meadows of watercress, lacking flavour, warmth or that feeling of satisfying fullness.

2   Because most people's efforts to lose weight come to nothing – or, in fact, result in weight gain, leading to those heart-sinking feelings of failure, hopelessness and an obligation to try again at something we've just learned we can't do.

Hardly surprising, then, that none of us like the idea. Losing weight tends to be an obligation rather than a choice, put upon us for health, social, medical, family or other reasons. Our conversation around weight loss is full of words about trying rather than doing, as if it's a given that we won't succeed.

First Time Fanny and the Failureville Bypass

If this is the first time in your life that you have had to consider losing weight then good on you – you're putting in the planning and preparation needed to do the job well, which makes you very likely to succeed. Don't let your enthusiasm be dampened by the endless moaning others do about how difficult it can be. Remember that obesity is a relatively new problem in society and we are only beginning to learn about how to deal with it. Yes, medical understanding of biology and metabolism has known for some time about what makes us put on weight, but because we are such complex creatures we need things like sociology, psychology and other areas of relevant expertise to catch up in order to find out why we do or don't succeed in our efforts. The psychology bit is what this book is about so you are at the right starting line.

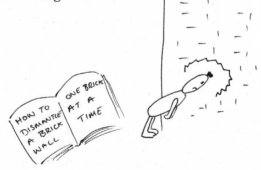

SOME PEOPLE MISUNDERSTAND THE CONCEPT OF
USING YOUR HEAD TO LOSE WEIGHT

The Comeback Kid

If you are a veteran of the weight-loss circuit then you may be coming to *Fabulous Jelly* feeling a little dubious. In fact, many dieters approach weight loss like it's going to jump up and bite them. In a way it does every time it doesn't go according to plan and leaves them feeling stupid, incompetent, weak or inferior to others. The Fabulous Jelly programme isn't the kind of plan where you have to take a deep breath and jump into something about as much fun as an ice bath. It's much more palatable than that. In fact, I shouldn't even say more 'palatable' – plain and simply it's just easier. The other good news for the comeback kid is that, whether you realise it or not, you have collected a mountain of information about what does and doesn't work for you.

Before going any further you need to take the time to find out which parts of any previous eating plan you've tried have worked a bit, a lot, or not at all, and why. Grab a pen and fill in the form on the next page and do really think about it (if you need more space copy the form onto a separate sheet). The Fabulous Jelly programme gives you a lot of flexibility and requires you to play around with a number of elements in your lifestyle. Because you have already tried other programmes you already know some of the things that work or don't work for you and what bits were just too difficult to stick to. Consciously identifying this information will really help to bring you success on the Fabulous Jelly programme and make you realise that it was elements of the plan that caused you to fall short of your goal. Yes, maybe one of those elements was willpower, but that's exactly what I'm talking about in this book. We only have a limited amount of willpower and it runs out. That is part of being human. It is not your fault. So if a diet demanded too much willpower then that was a fault in the programme, not you.

What You Can Learn from Previous Diets

	Diet 1	Diet 2	Diet 3	Diet 4	That' enoug
Diet name/label					
Planned duration					
Actual duration (how long you lasted)					

Description, e.g. set menu, counting points/calories/fat etc.				
Group/ Individual/ Online?				
Favourite foods allowed?				
Weight loss achieved				
Weight loss maintained				
Any new habits maintained, e.g. recipes, increased water intake, increased exercise, etc.				
Was exercise part of the plan?				
Level of difficulty (out of 10)				
Overall likeability (out of 10)				

GO BACK AND FILL IN THAT FORM!

YES, I TOO WOULD HAVE SKIPPED IT, BUT I'M TELLING YOU IT WILL ONLY TAKE A FEW MINUTES AND WILL HELP YOU TO SEE WHAT WORKED FOR YOU AND WHAT DIDN'T.

GRAB A PEN AND DO IT QUICKLY. IT WILL PROBABLY TAKE YOU ABOUT FOUR MINUTES.

Most readers will be in agreement that the whole weight-loss thing has become a bit of a chore, an ordeal, and a millstone round their necks. By doing the exercise above you should be able to take a few positives out of your past experiences with weight loss, by seeing what worked for you somewhat, a lot or not at all. You can use this information to avoid repeating past mistakes.

BE CAREFUL!

My husband is a kidney transplant recipient. When he was on dialysis I naturally wanted to provide him with as much nourishment as possible. I had read about juicing and thought this might be just the ticket for getting loads of nutrients into him. But I was wrong. What is healthy for one person is not necessarily so for another. A lot of fruit and vegetables have high concentrations of potassium and phosphates, something dialysis patients are trying to avoid. I discovered this just in time, but it was a valuable lesson in the definition of 'healthy'. Be careful.

By the way, grapefruit and cranberries are ones to watch if you are taking any medication as they can affect how some medicines are absorbed by the body. If you are on any medication, check with your doctor first before eating grapefruit or anything containing cranberries.

4

THE ENORMOUS BIG HUMDINGER OF AN ASK

Weight-loss programmes are awash with phrases like 'completely new you', 'transform yourself', 'never eat x again', 'change yourself forever', 'new life, new you' and so on. You can understand that this idea might appeal to anyone who's feeling like a big lump lacking in self-control. The promise of shedding all that physical and emotional weight sounds enticing. But what we all completely ignore is the role of the unconscious mind in all of this. We can knock ourselves out trying to get rid of excess weight but if we don't bring the unconscious mind on board we are creating unnecessary battles for ourselves that we just can't win. It's just too big an ask.

Keep in mind that your unconscious mind is the member-of-the-animal-kingdom-y part of our brain, running all the fantastically complex and phenomenally beautiful chemical interactions of the various systems necessary for our survival, such as the immune, hormonal, circulatory and respiratory systems of the body without any conscious input from us. Do you think that a 'whole new you' is likely to be acceptable to the keeper of your most primitive survival instincts? Of course not! No wonder you didn't have much success in the past! You've got to work with, not against, your natural instincts for self-protection, habit forming and love of the status quo which are programmed into your unconscious brain.

The unconscious (also called the subconscious) is all the information, memories, instincts, habits, values, beliefs, biases, learning, dreams, fears and absolutely everything we know and know how to do that we are not consciously aware of at any one moment. In essence, your subconscious is your essence. It is the sum of your genetics, history, environment and experience. It's who you are, what makes you you.

We have seen in a previous chapter that our brains like patterns, which are reflected in our behaviour as habits. When it can, the brain will tend to do *and think* the same way that it has previously. It's a bit like being set to autopilot unless we choose otherwise. By this I

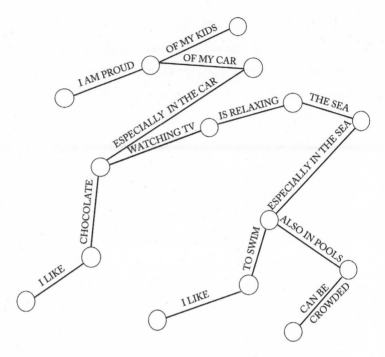

EVERY THOUGHT, FEELING AND BEHAVIOUR HAS
A CORRESPONDING NEURAL PATHWAY OF BRAIN
CELLS TALKING TO EACH OTHER. IN THIS EXAMPLE
THE PERSON MENTALLY LINKS CHOCOLATE WITH
LIKING, WITH BEING IN THE CAR AND WITH
WATCHING TV.

mean that unless we become aware of our tendency to think or act in a certain way, our brain will direct us to do what we have always done in the past. In biological terms everything we think and do has a corresponding physical set of neurons (nerve cells), communicating with each other by electrical and chemical messages. Although we have an estimated hundred billion neurons in the brain alone, let's pretend for simplicity that each letter of the alphabet is a brain cell (neuron). The pattern of B talking to K, talking to G, talking to F, talking to U might be the pattern of the thought 'I like football'. Another pattern involving K talking to Q, talking to D, talking to R, talking to T is the pattern corresponding to the recognition of water falling from the sky as being rain. Think how many of these patterns we must have in our brains!

A nice way to visualise these neuronal (nerve) connections is like a well-trodden path. Imagine you are standing at one side of a field of tall grass and I ask you to make your way to the other side of the field. The grass is above head height and you know that you are going to have to put a bit of effort into pushing your way through to the other side. You can go any way you want and will probably take the shortest route, and if you encounter obstacles you'll work your way around them.

The next day you come back to the same field and I again ask you to cross to the opposite side. You can go any route you choose, but having taken a look you see that the grass you pushed your way through yesterday is still slightly trodden down and would probably be your best bet. Sure enough this plan works and you arrive on the other side. The next day, the same task and guess what? The route you took on the previous two days is now a well trodden path and is definitely the path of least resistance. (On the fourth day you have the sense not to show up.)

This is roughly the way the neural pathways in your brain (and body) develop and the biological underpinning of habits occurs. It is also why practising anything makes you more likely to do it that way again next time. You are literally laying down a pathway that, through repetition, becomes the easiest path for your brain to fire off (activate) – on competition day, or indeed any other day of your life. And it's not just actions that have a corresponding neural pathway.

Sports psychology is a relatively new area of psychology. In the past much of what sports psychologists did was taking what we had already discovered in neuroscience and other areas of psychology, and adapting it for use in sport. However, as the field has developed and received more funding, researchers have discovered many things that are, in turn, relevant to weight loss.

Thinking, imagining and deeply held beliefs also arise from neurons making connections with each other throughout the whole body. In this era of professional psychology we are increasingly likely to hear professional athletes thanking their psychologist for the part they played in their success. Thinking a thought or imagining something happening 're-runs' the corresponding neural pathway. This action strengthens the links between the neurons involved, making the pathway stronger and thus making it even more likely that your brain will fire off that pattern again next time. As it's often put in text books: 'cells that fire together, wire together'.

On the playing field this can be good news. By the time you get to the top tier in any professional sport you are likely to already be doing the maximum amount of physical training that your body can take, and any more such training will actually work against you by depleting your energy and risking injury. So instead the sports stars turn to visualisation.

Using visualisation the person sees themselves carrying out a particular stroke, hit, kick, etc., with perfect technique. In doing this they are laying down – and reinforcing – the neuronal pathways that represent that action in the brain. If we go back to that pathway through the grass analogy we can see how treading down that tall grass again and again and again might make it easier and faster to pass through and make it the most obvious path to take through the grass. In much the same way, repeatedly visualising the perfect technique makes it more likely that the brain will fire that perfect technique neural pathway when it counts. These pathways aren't limited to the brain. In fact, if we were to hook a person up to the right equipment and get them to imagine themselves carrying out a movement, we would be able to see neural signals arriving at all the muscles involved in that movement. For example, if you were attached to the machine and imagined yourself moving your arm, we would see activity in the muscles of your arm – just not enough to actually move it. The more of the senses you throw in the more parts of the brain are involved in the pathway. For the athlete this might mean imagining the feeling of the racquet in their hand, or the feeling as they tap the end of the pool before turning, the sound of their teammates calling to them or the smell of other horses (or athletes!) in the arena.

So professional athletes *choose* what pathways they want to reinforce regarding their sport. When was the last time you checked in on your neural pathways?

THE 21-DAY MYTH

Many people will have heard it said that it takes twenty-one days for us to develop a new habit. Unfortunately this is a myth that seems to have arisen from confusion about the difference between getting used to something (known as habituation) and habit forming. In reality we all probably vary in how quickly we form a habit and the time required will also depend on the complexity and desirability of the behaviour we are trying to initiate. In one study, researchers who tried to create the simple habit of drinking a glass of water after breakfast took an average of sixty-six days to get a sense of the action being automatic.[3] When it comes to changing eating behaviours you are likely to find some are easier to change than others. Give yourself a lot longer than the mythical twenty-one days to change your eating habits and don't look at your diet as one habit; within it are a multitude of habits of various strengths and sizes.

Most of us never question how we think. We take our thoughts, views, beliefs and opinions as a given. Even if they are worse than useless we just swallow them all hook, line and sinker. But what if we had a choice? Would you *choose* to think the way you do about the world, yourself and other people? Would you *choose* to believe the things you do? Have you ever wondered …

ARE YOUR THOUGHTS, OPINIONS AND BELIEFS WORKING FOR YOU?

Are they useful? Are they getting you where you want to go? The chances are some are useful and some are not, but you probably don't know which ones are which because you've never spent time thinking about them. They just kind of are.

The problem with this is that it's a bit like choosing the house you're going to live in for the rest of your life or the person you're going to live with for the rest of your life by lottery. Would you be perfectly happy with that? The good news is you can choose which thoughts and attitudes are helpful and which might need changing or need to be dumped altogether. As I said before, some of these beliefs (known as 'Core Beliefs' in cognitive behavioural therapy-speak), are very unconscious and are difficult to challenge on your own – after all, it's hard not to agree with yourself! But let's take a look at some of the ones that spring to mind relatively easily. This will give you an idea of just how much muck we tend to gather over the course of our lifetimes without any conscious choice.

NOTE: If you suffer from depression or any psychiatric disorder your symptoms may make this exercise more difficult to do than it should be, so just skip this exercise for the moment. You might also want to discuss your weight-loss goals with a professional psychologist/psychiatrist or GP and find out how you can incorporate the Fabulous Jelly programme most easily into your life.

Draw a table like the one in the example overleaf on a piece of paper. In the left-hand column write some beliefs you have about yourself. Just let them flow; they can be positive and negative. Write them down as they come into your mind – don't try to edit them as this will only block the next one from coming. List as many beliefs about yourself as you can think of first. Then in the next column write down where you think you got each belief. And in the next column try to put in what age you were when you think you acquired this belief. In the next column give a percentage to represent to what extent this is an accurate description of you *as you are today*. And in the final column pay attention to the more negative beliefs about yourself that you have written down. Write down what evidence you have to the contrary.

Sample Table Examining Beliefs about Yourself

Belief	From where	Age started	Percentage accurate today	Contradictory evidence
I'm scatter-brained	Mum always said	10	30%	Revert to this when around my family and when I'm nervous/ stressed. Not true rest of time

Most people really enjoy this exercise since it can be a real eye-opener as to just how much of our beliefs were not ours to begin with, we just sort of adopted them without thinking about them. It can be really refreshing to suddenly remember that a particular negative belief came from a disgruntled teacher whose outbursts would nowadays land them in court, or a jealous sibling who said something hurtful once and never again but stung us enough to be remembered forever. What's even more surprising is the stuff we take on board that *was never said or meant.*

Communication is a very big subject; perhaps the most important thing to remember about it is this:

WHAT IS SAID ISN'T NECESSARILY WHAT IS UNDERSTOOD

In what is known as the 'Cocktail Party Effect' we are especially attuned to information that is – or that we think might be – about us. But sometimes we read between the lines and get the message completely confused. I used to give workshops on communications to transition-year students around the age of fifteen or sixteen. I often told them the following story:

Jack and Jill are brother and sister, aged sixteen and fifteen, respectively. One evening their mum and dad are having friends over for dinner and introduce the teenagers to their guests. Mum and Dad have read all the parenting books available and try to be as praising as possible as they introduce Jack.

'This is Jack. He has just got his school exam results back and we're really proud of how hard he worked,' says the mother, trying to praise the effort rather than the result like the books said.

While the guests subtly refill their glasses, anticipating a mind-numbingly dull evening, the parents continue, 'And this is Jill. She's just been picked to be captain of her basketball team. We're so proud of her.'

I then ask the students what they think Jill understands from this introduction. Without fail they tell me that Jill feels that her parents are insinuating that she is not academically gifted, and are just trying to get around the subject. It's amazing! In the story, Jill's parents made no mention of her academic abilities and focused purely on the positive, and yet all students 'read between the lines' of what is said with very negative consequences. This is not just true of young people. We all do it: we read between the lines and make inferences about what others say, arriving at sometimes completely inaccurate beliefs about ourselves that have nothing to do with what was said! Very often, we keep on believing these things for the rest of our lives. This can be especially true of things learned during moments of high emotion, like being ridiculed by a teacher, bullied by a classmate or being told off by a furious parent. The more emotional the moment, the faster it gets burned into memory. This makes sense in terms of our early evolution when things were really rotten and truly dangerous. In those days remembering facts like 'Camilla in cave 2B is psychotic' and 'the purple plant where we put out the bones is poisonous' could indeed have saved our lives.

In the Dock: Challenging the Thoughts You Didn't Know You Had

In the table below you are going to apply a version of the previous exercise to some of the beliefs that you hold about yourself and your weight. As before, you will first list them and then 'put them in the dock', i.e. take a fresh look to see how accurate they are now or ever were. Because we hold most of these beliefs unconsciously, we often never bring them to full conscious awareness and therefore never use our intelligent logical parts of our mind to test and challenge them. That's what this exercise is about. Start by just listing some beliefs that you have about yourself and your weight as statements in the left-hand column.

For example, did your sister tell you that you didn't fit into the dress because she wanted to wear it or she didn't want to be the only one it didn't fit. Or perhaps she was simply being a narky cow. Did your dad come out with sweeping statements about having a slow metabolism running through the family because it was easier for him to believe that that was why he was overweight?

Let all the beliefs and self-statements flow. You can then focus on anything particularly relating to your, or anyone else's, weight, shape, body, etc.

Here are some examples:

Some people are just lucky to be slim – they have good genes.

I'm big-boned/born big – my parents were overweight.

I have no sticking power – I always have short relationships too.

Anyone of a healthy weight is 'Skinny'.

I've no self-motivation.

I'm lazy.

This is what God wants for me.

All my family put on weight easily.

I like being the chubby, cheery type/the funny guy.

I hate that skinny uptight woman look.

Skinny women are control freaks.

I couldn't give up my boys' night.

My wife likes me 'cuddly'.

Thin people just look older faster.

I don't have time to lose weight now.

It's not my fault – it's because of my job … sitting at the desk all day … taking it in turns to get coffees and cakes at 11 … social lunches and business dinners.

I'm too wrecked to bother with dieting now.

I'm not going to put myself through the torture – I never last.

I hate the self-righteous skinny police.

I have the right to be any way I want.

I'd miss the hilarious chats I have with friends about our pathetic attempts at weight loss.

I've always been more the 'man friend' type rather than the romantic interest type of guy.

Beliefs About You and Your Weight in the Dock

Belief:	From whom/ where (frame):	When it began (approx. age):	Arguments for:	Arguments against:	Possible alternative belief:

Have You Been Selling Yourself a Pup?

Now that you have identified a few of the beauties that you've been living your life by, it may be dawning on you that we are not quite the free spirits we might fancy ourselves to be, but that, in fact, we live according to very deeply entrenched beliefs and values that act as guiding principles every day of our lives. Some of these stalwarts of the depths of the unconscious mind may be serving us well and don't need any updating (although it's always worth knowing them in case they work against us at some stage). However, if you feel as if you've been bashing your head against the proverbial brick wall when it comes to weight loss, the chances are these beliefs need their bottoms hauled out into the open to answer a few questions. You may then find that you are actually rather fond of their tiny little behinds as they bring you back to things Mum or Dad used to say at the dinner table etc. Look at it this way: this is not about cutting the apron strings so much as making sure they are not wrapped around your throat.

Frame

Taking each one in turn, take a look first at the 'Frame' or context where you learned the belief. Were you told to eat everything on your plate by a parent who grew up in poverty and whose own parents in turn struggled to put food on the table? In previous generations in Ireland, excess weight could identify someone as being wealthy and successful. Or perhaps you just liked the 'cuddliness' of a parent's tummy. Perhaps your Mum was always in the kitchen baking or cooking and gave you little treats as a means of showing you her love. Perhaps you knew someone who was slim built and stern and you began to associate slimness with narkiness or being unapproachable. Were you the chubby class joker? Maybe this role worked for you. Not too cool as to be unapproachable yet funny enough that everybody liked you so it worked well for you – and perhaps still does. Or maybe your whole family are/ were overweight. If so, you may well have a belief that you have a hormonal problem running in the family. This may, of course, be true, but, unless it has been identified in tests, it may be the case that it was much easier for one or both of your parents to accept the label of a medical condition rather than the fact that they have been feeding their children rubbish for far too long. In this case the 'frame' is an overweight parent who doesn't want to face the truth.

Evidence and Alternatives

Next we need to look at the evidence for and against the belief. It is OK to write down the evidence supporting a belief as otherwise it will just feel like a sneaky, guilty little niggle that will distract you from looking at the evidence against it. Remember, we are just trying to air the pros and cons of a belief and we may find that some of them are OK. We want to find a new, alternative possibility for ways of seeing things – a sort of 'working hypothesis'. This hypothesis must be somewhat acceptable to you at least in principle, and you can then go off and test it in your everyday life to see if it's a good/better/more accurate way of looking at things.

So write down: What is the evidence *for* this belief?

Next, what is the evidence *against* this belief?

Let's take a look at a few examples:

Belief: *I'm too wrecked to try to lose weight.*

For: *It is true to say I stay late at work most evenings and then take ages to get myself off the couch and into bed. My wife also works, so when I'm home I have to mind the kids so I can't get out for exercise.*

Against: *This is a case of false logic. Sounds like you probably are wrecked and I'm not going to pump out the usual stuff you already know about healthy eating and energy levels. This book is about the motivation to get started in the first place. The assumption hiding in the statement is that dieting takes time out of our day. More importantly it's a very sweeping statement (belief) that it takes a lot of time. Bringing this kind of assumption into your conscious awareness means that we can get a bit more accuracy into it. Weight loss doesn't have to take time out of your day – after all, all you need to do is eat less. Realistically, it does help if you could spare a bit of time for* *exercise, as it will speed up your weight loss, which in turn gives you the motivation to keep going. However, exercise isn't absolutely necessary. Could you find two periods of twenty minutes each week for exercise? Maybe, you don't feel you have the energy Monday to Friday but could you manage it on Saturday and Sunday? Admittedly, the health police will say this isn't enough to achieve weight loss or improve heart health, but that's not the point at the moment. Your goal here is to change that huge overriding, sweeping belief that you're too tired to lose weight. (You may also have a mental picture of yourself exercising that's just not pretty – we'll deal with that in the section dealing with exercise later on.)*

And then there's that bit that you know is coming that they show in all those healthy eating programmes on television: hours upon hours of endless vegetable chopping. The good news is that this isn't a prerequisite for weight loss either (although it does help). I'll deal with this issue in the next chapter but, for the moment, just consider the possibility that all that you need to do is to change some of the contents of your shopping basket.

Alternative: *Would you now be willing to consider the possibility that weight loss doesn't have to take time out of your day or demand loads of energy from you? Again,* *all we are looking for here is a possibility. You can investigate yourself to find if this is actually true and is a more accurate way of looking at things.*

Let's take a look at another belief:

Belief: *I NEVER stick to diets. FACT!*

For: *In the past not once did I stick to the eating plan devised for me/that I devised to lose weight. I always stopped before I planned to.*

Against: *Wouldn't it be more accurate to say 'I have never stuck to a diet* so far'? *The belief smacks of all-or-nothing thinking (see Chapter 1), but by changing it to this alternative we instantly make it:*

1. *More accurate*

2. *Less rigid*

3. *Less fortune-telling about the future*

It doesn't take much analysis to see that the insinuation in this belief is 'I'm going to fail next time too, so why bother?'

In this case it may not be possible to deny that you stopped the diet earlier than you planned, but we may (or may not) be able to get a few positives out of some careful investigation – or at the very least some additional information. Go back to the table in chapter 3 to establish what worked and what didn't work on your previous diets.

Alternative: *Now we need to look for a potential candidate for a new belief and you can later decide whether it is more useful or not. You could say: 'I have never stuck to a diet so far, but I did learn that set menu plans don't suit me or my biggest difficulty is (x) and I need to look at ways of getting around this problem.' Now we have a far more accurate statement that makes it obvious where you need extra help.*

It's really important that your new alternative potential beliefs aren't so overly positive and rosy that you simply don't believe them. Remember these are beliefs that will become unconscious to you in the future if they are acceptable to you, but they won't work if you don't believe them 'in your heart of hearts'.

In the Dock

Continue down through your list of beliefs and carry out the same steps for each one:

1 Identify the frame – can you pinpoint where you got this belief?

2 Identify (if you can) when you started to believe this statement to be true. Doing this can often highlight just how out-of-date this belief really is.

3 List the arguments (if any) that support the belief.

4 List the evidence against this belief.

5 Write a *realistic* potential alternative belief that you can use as a hypothesis to be tested, to see if it is more accurate.

5

Prostrate Yourself Before Your Unconscious Mind and Start Grovelling

So now you have finally figured out who's boss – and it isn't you. Your previous attempts at weight loss were like a cat with a mouse in its sights allowing the mouse to escape a little just because it enjoys catching it again. You were the mouse. Well at least now you know who you need to make your case to when it comes to your weight loss.

But know this. Your unconscious mind doesn't want to change. It's full of survival instincts – to suckle, sleep, have sex and eat; neural pathways of habit and clever protective mechanisms. It's got the fight or flight response in there too, in case of lion attacks, but it isn't quite up to speed with the obesity epidemic. It's a happy camper with the way things are and a big fan of the status quo. It's what makes you human but is the bit of the brain that has most in common with the animal kingdom. The bit that emerged first in our evolution. It's not interested in good manners or what others think other than with the little caveat that there's safety in numbers – think herd mentality. As far as your unconscious mind is concerned, your excess layers of adipose (fat) are like the most exquisite fur coat with a handy little survival kit in the inside pocket in case of emergency or famine.

To change your weight you need to ask permission. You need to keep in mind everything you have learned in the previous chapter about the guiding beliefs and values that your unconscious holds regarding every-thing to do with fat, weight, your figure, your ability to change, beliefs about whether or not you have choices, etc. By carrying out the exercises related to these beliefs you have begun to inject a little bit of doubt as to their validity, but these are still what you need to keep in mind as you make your case.

Of course, there is no actual presentation to the unconscious. That bit is metaphorical. But the rest is not. If you want to feel like you have a real fighting chance with any weight-loss programme, you need to feel in your 'heart of hearts' that it sits right with you. You need to honestly *believe* that it takes you, and all your strengths and weaknesses, into consideration. How many previous programmes felt like this? Did you feel madly, urgently determined and revved up when starting previous eating programmes? Did you need this unusual surge of motivation to get you started? If so, you were probably doomed from the start. How many of us have felt this way on the first of January – or a birthday or anniversary, or just another Monday – but the motivation had left us high and dry by the next day? If you needed this much 'revving up', your 'heart of hearts' could have told you it wasn't going to last.

As you proceed through this book I hope that you will begin to learn to observe your own thoughts: to understand them as optional ways of seeing things and to identify what sincerely 'sits right' with you as you are now, rather than some ideal version of you. At the start of any new eating programme ask yourself if you really believe that the programme is doable for you. Is it realistic? Does it take your lifestyle into account and allow you enough flexibility? Have a look through its blurb and see if you can identify any of the extremes of thinking that we have spoken about.

Beware of all-or-nothing statements, such as:

- Never eat x again

- Look forward to a whole new you

- Let go of …

- Change your lifestyle …

You just don't have to work that hard – and we don't want a whole new you.

THE MOST ESSENTIAL POINT IN ALL OF THE FABULOUS JELLY PROGRAMME IS THIS:

YOU NEED TO WORK WITH, NOT AGAINST, YOUR UNCONSCIOUS MIND AND ALL ITS INSTINCTS TO AVOID CHANGES THAT IT THINKS MIGHT BE DANGEROUS TO YOUR EXISTENCE – LIKE DIETS!

6

THE FABULOUS JELLY PROGRAMME

STEP UP TO THE PLATE!
HELL, ROLL AROUND IN IT!
HAVE YOUR CAKE – AND EAT IT!

The Fabulous Jelly programme is really a set of guidelines to help you find what will work for you. You can use them in conjunction with an eating plan devised by a nutritionist if you like or simply follow the guidelines alone. As I've said before, I am not a nutritionist and nowhere here do I offer specific details about nutrition. There are thousands of books and websites on the topic for you to refer to if you need more information.

To keep the unconscious happy we need to be careful not to change too much too quickly, as that would be an assault on who we are and who we have been all our adult lives. We also need to see (show the unconscious) results as soon as possible, as this is a huge motivator to keep going. If we see weight loss, our efforts are no longer a pointless sacrifice but, instead, a fair give and take relationship, similar to paying over money and receiving a product in return. This is perfectly just and appeals to our unconscious. It's like the difference between a parent instructing a child to pick up a piece of someone else's litter and put it in the bin 'because it's the right thing to do for the community' and telling the child they will get a bar of chocolate for doing it. The first is asking the child to understand the intangible, abstract ideas of 'right' and 'community', which is difficult (but not wrong), compared to the very logical lesson of exchange of effort for reward.

So here it is: Introducing the easy does it, step-up-to-the-plate-and-crawl-in-style Fabulous Jelly weight-loss programme that has helped me to lose over two stone in weight – and keep it off.

On it you are going to be …
1 Keeping
2 Tweaking and swapping
3 Diarying
4 Exercising

... to glorious abandon while losing weight almost painlessly.

Because everyone is different and some people will only need to identify one or two bad habits, while others will find it faster to list their good eating habits, you will need to make many of your own judgements in terms of quantities and shout 'foul' when you're not being honest with yourself. But there is no big start day with fanfare. You can start right now making some mild (relatively) painless changes that will mean that you will go to bed tonight having taken in less calories and fat than you would have had you not got the ball rolling gently. And because there is no 'giving up' involved there is also no need for any 'last time' dashes to the shop to have the last ever taste of your favourite bar of chocolate, crisps, sausage rolls or take-away. Doesn't that sound like a good proposition?

What I can tell you though, from experience, is that the more effort you put into the programme the quicker you will get results. The quicker you see results the more you want to protect them and the easier all the tweaking becomes and the more creative you get in terms of balancing out your energy intake and output. As I do not give any nutritional information you will need to look after this issue as soon as you can, but you will still be able to use the guiding principles outlined here. If you were mentally ready to follow a perfectly nutritionally balanced diet you wouldn't be reading this book.

WEIGHING IN

Many readers will be familiar with the traditional advice to avoid weighing themselves more than once a week. The logic behind this advice was that our weight will naturally fluctuate with hormonal variations and so we might be de-motivated if we see that our weight has gone up before the effects of our weight-loss efforts have had time to kick in.

However, I ignored this advice. I knew that as I was developing my own eating guidelines I needed more immediate feedback on my efforts. If I was kidding myself the scales would not lie. I am a big girl and able to take the odd disappointment when my weight increased very slightly, but I also knew full well when trying to blame hormonal changes was not going to cut the mustard. Overeaters can do a whole lot of damage in a week – especially when they are in that 'I've started (the week badly) so I'll finish (the week badly)' sort of mood.

Recent research is, in fact, backing up the daily weigh-in strategy. Like keeping a food diary, stepping on the scales every day helps us to monitor ourselves and get fast, and hopefully positive, feedback.

Guideline No. 1: Identify Your Keepers

What is it that you think you just can't stop eating? Is there something that you crave – perhaps at a particular time of day? It might be a particular bar of chocolate on your way home from work – or just chocolate in general. Perhaps you eat at least one bar every day of the week and just can't summon up the strength not to buy it. Or maybe it's some other type of sweets, or a daily muffin, scone and jam or take-away. Maybe it's having a beer every night or a breakfast roll from the petrol station, complete with sausages, bacon and the works. At the time I started the Fabulous Jelly programme I had got into the habit of eating a bar of chocolate almost every day. And because I was in that all-or-nothing frame of mind and was disgusted with myself for not being able to get my act together enough to stop the chocolate habit, I also just generally ate too much. Not absolutely terrible stuff, mostly just far too much bread. But too much of anything will pile on the weight. The chances are, if you are feeling angry enough with yourself to be reading this you are probably on the same train. And so you pile the extra helping on your dinner plate, say 'yes' to the slice of cake with coffee and/or find yourself giving yourself a lot of 'little treats' throughout the week.

You need to decide what you really can't change for the time being. If you really can't stop yourself stopping at the shop for chocolate on your way home from work (and you've tried willpower and taking a different route home), then how about trading down to another bar that is still chocolate? Something that still deals with the craving but is not your usual choice. For example, could you choose a Curly Wurly bar instead of a bar of Dairy Milk or a Snickers? Put a little bit of thought into what you could change to that would reduce the fat and calories. How about some of the boiled sweets which have become so popular again lately and are readily available in tubs or traditional paper bags? If you try them you will probably find that they deal with the craving enough to get you over that moment in your day that you associate with the chocolate. You are also likely to find that there are only so many boiled sweets you can eat so you won't eat as many of them as you might think.

People often talk about their cravings as if a particular bar/item has a hold over them. Swapping to another type of sweet deals with the sugar craving (which will eventually have to be dealt with in a healthier manner) while also breaking the feeling of helplessness. It acts as an acceptable consolation prize, giving a lesser reward, which in turn makes cutting this down or out at a later point much easier to do. It also is often more acceptable than just not stopping at the shop at all (again a better option), although you will aim for this at a later date. For some people stopping at the shop and not buying anything is just too big an ask to begin with. Even the journey to the shop has become part of the pleasure ritual.

Changing to an alternative but lesser pleasure is key in identifying your most suitable 'Keepers'. (By Keepers I mean something that is still enjoyable but lesser in terms of fat/sugar/calorie content.) What would you be willing to have instead that would be acceptable to you? Even three plain biscuits with your evening cup of tea would be a better option than most bars of chocolate – especially if you are making healthy swaps and tweaks with the rest of your diet.

If crisps are your thing these can be your Keepers on the programme if you need them. However, take a look at all the baked varieties. Would they be as delicious to you as your favourite brand? Probably not. But at least you're not being asked to give them up completely. You can either decide you really want to keep them but will be extra careful with the rest of your eating, or you can choose the healthier varieties that will deal with the craving but lessen the reward enough to make them easier to wean yourself off if you need to at a later date. Try it. You will find that your craving for your full-fat favourite will be gone once you have had the lighter type. Again, it's just enough to do the trick and this is what you are looking for, for the moment.

The key to choosing your Keepers is to find something that will be acceptable to you as a trade-off to replace or reduce your unhealthy favourite foods without much effort. It might be just less of that something, perhaps kept until after your evening meal if you think that will be enough of a motivator to keep you going throughout the day. I know someone who avoids the bread basket, heavy sauces and desserts when eating out by having a packet of wine gums in her handbag which she then allows herself to have with a cup of tea when she gets home. Ideal? No, it would be better if she didn't have the sugar just before getting into bed, but as a trade-off for all the extra calories she could have consumed during the meal it's perfect for the moment. If you find you can't resist the cheese board when eating out you might find that allowing yourself one or two crackers without the cheese is enough to stop you sampling everything on offer. Or maybe just making sure you have a cup of coffee in your hand while the cheese board is on the table will be enough to keep your hands occupied and prevent 'nibble wander'.

If your favourite food is associated with a place, such as a coffee shop you pass every day on the way to work, or a stall in the park where you bring your children, you could choose to change to a different item to wean yourself off the demon 'treat'. This will allow you to weaken the associations in your mind between the place and reward without too much willpower being required. This way you are not trying to break down all the pieces of the association as it is mapped out in your brain, involving the journey to the place, the place itself, the item of food and, of course, all the other details of the experience that your brain takes in unconsciously without your conscious awareness.

When choosing your Keepers do your best to choose a different food rather than just less of the same, as this will break the associations you have with that food. When it comes to people who have been in the habit of overeating there is an element of a 'stick-something-in-my-mouth' compulsion whether we realise it or not – and usually that something is mostly sugar in some form or another. We are all aware of the dangers of sugar, but many don't realise that the whole experience of the preparation and eating (even scoffing) becomes a set piece of behaviour; it may be easier to prise yourself away from some of it rather than all of it at once. As you follow the rest of the Fabulous Jelly programme you'll be feeling much more ready – in fact eager – to take another step away from old habits. Remember, these habits are often habits of a lifetime – give yourself time!

In my case the chocolate had to go. Every time I ate a bar of chocolate I felt annoyed with myself. It made me feel slobby. I also knew it had become a trigger for me in terms of the rest of my daily diet. In true all-or-nothing style when I was eating chocolate it was like a signal to me to not bother with the rest of my eating. Had I been able to allow myself *a little* chocolate without guilt I could have taken it to be my Keeper and used it as a little reward for eating well the remainder of the day or week. But I know me and I don't do 'a little chocolate/a square or two'. It just had to go.

For me the substitute was allowing myself biscuits at the end of the day with a cup of tea. I also used to buy jellies or wine gums and had them when I really felt I wanted them. Obviously jellies are very high in sugar and not even a medium-term good idea. But they worked a treat. I never loved jellies so they were never going to be something I would go overboard on. They just ticked a box in the times that I might otherwise have eaten chocolate. They were so sweet that I would only ever eat a few and after about a month I had all but forgotten about them.

Remember, this is not about giving yourself permission to have a sugar fest. This is a weaning process where you are cutting down on the bad stuff, upping the good stuff and giving your unconscious some really positive feedback about making changes by achieving weight loss way in excess of the few pounds you may naturally fluctuate. Your overall calorific intake should be less than it was before you started Fabulous Jelly.

All you are doing here is making changes gradually, while achieving weight loss worth protecting quickly enough to keep you motivated. If you are kidding yourself the scales will let you know very quickly.

GIVE UP GIVING UP STUFF – AND GIVING UP, TOO!

Fabulous Jelly is not about asking you to give up anything completely or forever. As you have probably learned by now those sorts of plans tend to come to an unhappy end with you kicking yourself for failing. Instead you are looking for healthier alternatives or 'swaps' while keeping something for yourself that ticks that 'treat' box – your Keepers.

When I swapped chocolate for jellies I didn't make any plans for how long I would keep up the swap yet I haven't eaten a bar of chocolate in nearly a year. I'm sure I will again some time – I just knew it had become a habit and I needed to swap it for something else for the time being.

If you try to give up sweets you will find that your cravings will dissipate in forty-eight hours. Of course this is the best plan of action. However, I am presuming here that you have already tried this and not been able to resist temptation or just cannot find the willpower to even try. That's why we are playing the negotiation game for the moment.

Guideline No. 2: Swapping and Tweaking – Targeting Your Low-Hanging Fruit

'Low-hanging fruit' is business-guru terminology for picking off the easy changes first. In the case of business it usually means starting with the changes that are likely to save the company money with little effort or pain. It's the equivalent of eye-level-and-below dusting in the housework world, or starting your work day by accepting invitations in your inbox to link or befriend: just doing the easy bits first.

There are three basic areas that you need to focus your swapping or tweaking on. The first is in reducing the amount of carbohydrates you take in, the second and related one is increasing the amount of vegetables. The third is a more general one: to be prepared when temptation strikes and to have an alternative available.

YOUR CARBOHYDRATES ARE FIRST TARGET ON YOUR LIST

If you are overweight the chances are you are eating too many carbohydrates. Although vegetables and fruit contain some carbohydrate, we could probably safely guess that these are not your problem. Expert views vary over just how many carbs we should be eating and whether cutting them almost completely out of your diet is healthy. However, there is probably plenty of room for manoeuvring in terms of your carb intake before you need to worry about this.

The fact is you probably need to cut down your carbs *a lot*.

Of course, as I am not a dietician and do not know your eating regime, the degree to which you do this is up to you and you may need to experiment a little until you find the right balance between keeping up your energy levels and taking in far more calories than you are burning.

Bread, pasta, rice and potatoes are full of calories. Yes they contain energy and if you eat the more wholegrain versions of bread and pasta they will balance your sugar levels, but you don't need nearly as much of them as you are probably eating. If you did you wouldn't have put on weight. Many women serve themselves up the same portion of pasta or potatoes as they give to their male partners even though a man will burn more calories, even asleep, than a woman will. You do not need all this excess stodge in your stomach. Have you seen flour and water – the ingredients of pasta – used as wallpaper paste? Try doing this yourself using tissue or a piece of paper instead of the wallpaper (unless of course you actually need a bit of DIY to be done, in which case you'll have a blast) and it might just be enough to change your view of white pasta as a nutritious food.

Bread is another problem area. Not that it is bad in and of itself, but a huge number of people who are overweight just eat too much of it. It also tends to make you lazy about what else you eat as it's very easy to just stick any old spread or processed meat on top. Many people say that they simply couldn't give up bread. You don't have to. But you do need to look at your overall carb intake and reduce it a lot.

The jury is also out on whether the time of day you eat your calories matters in managing your weight. Does it matter if you eat your carbs with your evening meal? Is it better to skip carbs after lunchtime? The experts disagree. Find out for yourself. If you eat carbs with your dinner you are likely to see it on the scales if you weigh yourself the next day. This doesn't necessarily mean you have put on fat but only that the meal, or at least some of it, is still in your gut.

Remember you are making some temporary trade-offs for your Keepers. If you have generally already eaten some carbs during the day and you also want to have your Keepers then you are out of luck. You will have to skip the carbs for dinner and instead pile your plate high with vegetables. It's one or the other. (More on vegetables shortly.) You will, in fact, probably find it easier to cut the carbs in your evening meal if you know you have your Keeper treat to look forward to.

I also thought I couldn't do without bread. I never made the decision to cut it out almost completely, but I did choose to think of things to eat for lunch other than the inevitable sandwich. I have always made homemade soups of various varieties, so when I stopped eating sandwiches soup seemed like an obvious alternative. I also realised that throwing together a salad takes about as long as making a sandwich. Even though washed and bagged lettuce is a good bit more expensive than a head of lettuce, many people will find it's well worth the extra money to save time in their busy lifestyles. Throw in a couple of tomatoes, maybe some roasted red peppers from a jar (unless you have time to roast them yourself), maybe some stuffed olives, kale, gherkins, sundried tomatoes, tuna, a tiny bit of smoked sundried tomato pesto, or boiled or poached egg and/or a good salad dressing. Absolutely delicious! Salad doesn't have to mean 1980s' style lettuce, tomato and cucumber.

By the way, I recently bought a little set for poaching eggs in the microwave. Although I rather miss chasing bits of my egg around the saucepan of boiling water, the poaching plate means that I can time my egg to cook to precisely the way I like it and go off to do something else while it's cooking. It's very handy and an easy way of adding a bit of protein to a salad – not to mention heat, which tends to make a meal more satisfying.

YOU NEED TO EAT MORE VEGGIES

What vegetables do you like? How many different types of vegetables do you eat over the course of a week? How many different ways are they prepared? To the left and right of your pork chop does not count as two ways here. How many different colours of vegetables do you eat and are any of them eaten raw?

THE SALAD DRESSING IS IMPORTANT

Now there's something I never thought I'd say! Next time you are shopping take a look at the enormous variety of dressings available and compare the labels. While there are some that have a massive sugar and fat content and need to be avoided, there are loads of varieties that will absolutely make your salad a proper and delicious meal. Brilliant if you can choose a low-fat option such as the Weight Watchers or similar range. If not, keep in mind that the more liquidy vinaigrette-style dressings are often lower in fat than the thick-running dressings. Alternatively you might want to make your own dressing or simply use vinegar, salt, pepper and some lemon juice. The important point is that if you are going to start eating a whole lot more salads (warm and cold) the salad dressing becomes far more important on your shopping list than it may have been previously, so don't just skim past this section: decide what you prefer, buy or make it immediately, and start using it today.

Focusing on these few questions can help to get us out of the rut of 'same ol' same ol''. Remember that we are all creatures of habit and will return to things that give us comfort, even unconsciously. So it may be that you are serving up many of the same vegetables that your mother cooked for you, or perhaps cooking them the same way, which in Irish terms often means boiled to oblivion so that they haven't a trace of nutrients left in them.

FROZEN VEG. ARE THE NEW AVOCADO!

The good news is many frozen vegetables contain more of their nutrients than non-frozen because the freezing process locks in the goodness whereas non-frozen vegetables are continuously losing their nutritional value while they make the journey from field to fridge. So if, like me, you can't bear avocados and are fed up with hearing about how many avocados you should be eating you will be delighted to hear that there are lots of other ways to get your nutrients. True – they don't contain all the good types of fat that avocados do, but at least you are upping your nutrition from your starting point.

By the way, current knowledge suggests that tinned tomatoes could actually be considered a 'super food' as they're packed with nutrients and are actually even more nutritious than fresh tomatoes. However, the same doesn't apply to all vegetables so choose frozen not tinned for all other vegetables when not buying fresh.

Upping your vegetable intake will really help you to reduce your carbohydrates by helping to fill you up and becoming the 'bulk' item on your plate. Where before you may have piled mince on a plate of spaghetti or a chilli con carne sauce on top of a baked potato, you can now use mostly vegetables to provide that feeling of fullness. As they are mostly water you will stop gaining weight at *every single* dinner you eat as you have probably been doing for many years by piling on the carbs and not burning off the calories (calories = energy).

If your heart sinks at the prospect of eating a lot more vegetables don't worry. You just need to see how vegetables can be absolutely delicious – it just depends on how they are prepared and served. If you're unconvinced, google 'boring vegetables' for ideas.

Think of vegetables for dinner. What is the first visual that comes into your head? What feeling do you get? If it's a picture of a mound of sloppy nondescript watery sludge that's supposed to be rata-touille, or an image of peas beside a piece of meat then you really, really need to take a bit of time shopping around for new ideas on how to make vegetables deli-cious. Simple changes can completely change how you view them. For example, you may have eaten carrots chopped in circular slices for the last twenty years, or French beans that do little to inspire. In such instances your image of vegetables as dull would be absolutely spot on. However, if you toss a tiny bit of low-fat spread over some boiled sliced carrots with a splash of orange juice, pinch of salt and some ground ginger (if you like it), carrots might even begin to move centre stage on your dinner plate. Or toss them in a little honey and roast them.

Boring French beans are a thousand times nicer served sprinkled with toasted almonds. These are the kinds of things that you may not already have in your kitchen cupboards, but once you've bought a bag of sliced almonds they will last you a good while and will make you feel just *un peu* chef-like! Sprinkle them through the French beans and, if you like, add in a little bit of one of those low-fat spreads.

Many vegetables don't have much of a flavour, so

finding easy and fast ways to make them appetising is crucial. Tinned tomatoes, stock cubes, curry powder, chilli powder, mustard, paprika, Worcester sauce, soy sauce, garlic and onions will be your best friends in this regard. It's so important to be realistic about what you will and won't do, so if you think you won't have it in you to chop some fresh garlic then you can buy bags of pre-chopped garlic in many supermarkets (under cover of darkness to hide your shame!). Alternatively you could just chop more than you need on one evening and stick it in a container in the freezer. You can also buy a garlic press that holds garlic and can be stored in the fridge until you are ready to press it, much like a pepper mill.

If you have been struggling with trying to find the motivation to start losing weight then there is no point looking at complicated recipes. You will be better off starting with things that you can bung in the saucepan or oven, just as quickly as you threw potatoes, pasta or rice in hot water up until now.

Roasting bags will become your best friend. You can simply throw your chopped meat and chopped vegetables into these little clear plastic bags, add some herbs and seasoning and throw them in the oven where they will cook in their own juices, never dry out and produce a really healthy meal without even a mention of the d**t word.

If you like those packs of frozen broccoli, carrot and cauliflower mixes then brilliant – personally I think you are a saint to eat them. No wonder you want carbs. Take a look at the newer style of frozen vegetable mixes – some of them are absolutely delicious. Oriental, Mediterranean and Mexican style vegetable mixes are a brilliant way of 'interesting-up' your meal and will make it far more likely that you will be happy to pile them on your plate. Just make sure to take a look at the label, as once the manufacturers start making mixtures they can often sneak in extra fats. Don't confuse the frozen vegetable mixtures that I'm talking about with the 'rice and a few escaped vegetables thrown in' type mixtures – these are of course, mainly carbohydrates.

I have focused on frozen vegetables in this section because I think they are given too little attention in most diet and cookery books and also because of their obvious ease. However, of course, most of us have some days that we need to grab something from the freezer, and other days when we want to put a bit more effort into preparing our meal and use more fresh ingredients. You will probably find that as you lose weight you will take more interest in what you are eating and will take more time to prepare something really nice rather than grabbing anything and sticking it in your mouth.

Once you have lost weight you will happily put effort into protecting that weight loss. You will find it much easier to forego whatever rubbish is still lurking around your kitchen because you are delighted with yourself and because you can still look forward to your Keepers. It becomes much more about swapping than sacrificing and therefore doesn't require the will-power that is needed for so many weight-loss plans. Remember: we are 'enticing' the unconscious mind to come with us in 'trying out' weight loss. We are doing this by making small, relatively unchallenging changes and keeping things that we couldn't yet part with (our Keepers), while also delivering the positive rein-forcement of weight loss. We are coaxing our minds towards changing the habits of a lifetime.

BE PREPARED FOR THOSE 'STICK-ANYTHING-IN-MY-MOUTH' MOMENTS

If you are overweight you probably have developed a habit of sticking something in your mouth during mental downtimes. By this I mean those times when maybe your concentration has gone; for example, when working on something at the desk. (Try writing a book and you will know what I'm talking about!) These might include:

- arriving home

- office break time

- in the car

- when the children have gone to bed

- while cooking.

All of these daily events are very common trigger times for snacking and you need to put a bit of thought into how you will deal with them.

In the medium to long term you will want to get rid of the associations between these times and eating, but for the moment we are trying to wean you off the habit gently. Remember this kind of eating is a habit stored in the unconscious as a 'pathway' in the brain. Attempting to stop all of these habits at once may be too big an 'ask' and something that you might only do at the start of a new diet when you're feeling virtuous.

You need to make changes more gradually as this is less of a challenge to the way your brain is 'wired' and will allow you to keep up your motivation for longer.

Having a visual of what is actually happening in your brain might help you to appreciate just how important this is:

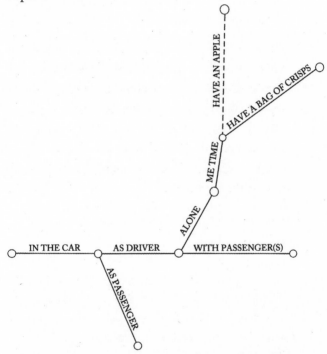

THIS PERSON HAS DEVELOPED NEURAL CONNECTIONS IN THE BRAIN BETWEEN 'IN THE CAR', 'AS DRIVER', 'ALONE', 'ME TIME' AND 'HAVE A BAG OF CRISPS', BUT ONLY TENTATIVE CONNECTIONS WITH 'HAVE AN APPLE' WHICH NEEDS TO BE REPEATED TO BE STRENGTHENED.

So what changes do you think would be realistic for you? Keep in mind that there are many elements within each habit. Take eating in the car for example. Within this habit these elements might include:

1 Sitting in driver's seat. (You probably don't have the same urge to eat as a passenger in a car. If you do it's another habit.)

2 After settling yourself into the seat, putting on your belt, etc., or after leaving the kids at school/finishing a meeting/spending a long time in the car. (If you find that you tend to snack in the car after coming out of a shop/petrol station, the association you need to work on may be buying snacks when surrounded by them in a shop, rather than eating in the car.)

3 Choosing the same snack each time.

4 Whether you buy the item or bring it with you from home.

5 The particular time of day or week. Maybe it's associated with a long(ish) drive somewhere or after doing the weekly grocery shop.

6 Whether there is someone else in the car with you. Is it a 'me-time treat' – or maybe you make it treat time for you and all the kids?

From a brain point of view all of these factors are

linked together to build your habit by connecting neurons. So one person's habit might link 'being alone' with 'refuelling at petrol station' with 'bar of X' with 'putting chocolate in mouth'. Someone else's habit might involve 'collecting kids from soccer' with 'passing chipper on way home' with 'smell of chips in chipper' with 'sensation of biting into a hot chip'.

In these examples it may be unrealistic to suggest that you avoid a particular petrol station or route home. But could you try to change to buying something less unhealthy, such as one or two pieces of fruit? Of course, this takes some self-control, but people often find that the fruit is enough to meet the desire to put something in their mouth. It probably won't taste as delicious as the chocolate/chips, but it is just enough to satisfy the putting something in your mouth bit of the habit while also starting to 'unhook' the habit from chocolate/chips. Importantly, giving yourself the lesser reward of a slightly smaller sugar hit will start to weaken the habit. It would also be possible to change to a different type of treat that you don't crave, but this should be used for only a short period in order to make the initial break with whatever you normally buy. Perhaps you could treat yourself to a magazine to read later for some down time and a water ice-type ice pop can be a sufficiently refreshing substitute for the more calorie-laden varieties of ice cream on a hot day.

Preparation is key: It's a good idea to have a bag of apples, easy peel mandarin oranges or any other fruit you like with you in the car, along with a small bag for cores, peel or whatever and some wipes. Once you have set this up in the car you are sorted and the new behaviour becomes far easier. The chances of someone sitting with the smell of the kids' chips in the car while they drive to find a shop that sells fruit is small. Sugar-free mints or gum might be enough to meet the urge to put something in your mouth just as well. Whatever you choose, be prepared!

Remember: You have your Keeper(s) to look forward to so this should be enough enticement to keep you away from other temptations. For this reason, saving your Keeper(s) until later in the day is usually helpful.

POSSIBLE SWAPS AND TWEAKS FOR WHEN YOU COME IN THE DOOR STARVING

- Raw carrots with hummus – so delicious you won't mind having to wash a carrot or two, and once you have a vegetable peeler easily to hand it's fast food

- Home-made soup (the weight-loss hero) – stick a bowl of soup in the microwave

- Fruit – preferably pre-peeled, chopped, etc. where necessary, or you won't eat it

- Celery and home-made salsa (pre-made at the weekend)

- Fizzy water – apparently not quite as healthy as the non-fizzy stuff but frankly at this stage that's like telling a beach donkey that the going will be soft underfoot at the Galway races this weekend – irrelevant. Try it as an alternative to fizzy drinks, cola, etc.

- Slices of turkey, maybe drizzled with a little pesto and rolled up

- Sliced smoked salmon (if it isn't pre-sliced you probably won't bother going through the mess of slicing it) drizzled with some lemon juice and rolled up

Throughout the whole Fabulous Jelly programme you are trying to gradually undo bad eating habits. Most eating programmes demand that you give up all your bad habits from the start. This is why getting started on such programmes brings on the 'all-or-nothing' thinking that we spoke about before. You're going to be 'really good ... starting tomorrow' so you allow yourself anything and everything you want before you get started. And possibly you do well for a while. But if you are reading this you know that extreme strategies take mental effort that is hard to keep up. This is why the Fabulous Jelly programme works with, not against, your lifelong habits. You are reducing the reward (usually sugar or fat) that kept them going so that the habit weakens and will be later replaced by a healthier alternative. If you can just stop doing whatever unhealthy habit(s) you have, go do it now!

While making some gradual changes you will be achieving weight loss by cutting down your intake of carbohydrates *a lot*, because if you are overweight it is likely that you are eating too many of them. Meantime you have the trade-off of your Keepers – a *LESSER* amount of those items you just couldn't give up yet. Most of the sensory and psychological pleasure of your take-away or other food 'treat' comes from the associations with perhaps a weekend night, an evening off cooking, eating on the couch, the heat, smell and strong flavours of the food, etc. You don't have to get rid of all of these pleasures or all parts of the ritual. It's really a matter of finding a healthier way of doing the same thing. In this regard the following cannot be overstated enough:

PREPARATION IS EVERYTHING

If you know you will be having a glass of wine or a beer with your partner or friend at home tomorrow evening and normally have a few nibbles with your drinks, then put a bit of thought into it the evening before. Get some carrots/celery/olives/very low-fat crisps into the house even if that means going out of your way to get them. Make up a quick salsa and make or buy some hummus or whatever healthier alternative nibbles you fancy. If you will be meeting at a bar that normally provides plates of peanuts or where you normally buy salty things like peanuts, then have a bag of something similar but lighter before you get there, such as salt and vinegar rice cakes. You won't stop liking peanuts, but you will have taken away your craving for something salty that drinking alcohol can often cause and you should have no problem avoiding the calorie- and fat-laden nuts and crisps at the bar.

BEST TAKE-AWAY ALTERNATIVE

The ritual is part of the habit here so if you usually heat plates in the oven while waiting for a take-away delivery then continue to do the same. If you lay a tray to take it in front of the TV then do it. (I won't repeat all the stuff about how many extra calories people consume if eating mindlessly in front of the TV, as you probably already know this and that you will need to work on it at some stage.)

You could choose to buy one of those calorie-controlled frozen meals such as spaghetti carbonara or chicken curry. You could also quickly heat up some tasty frozen vegetables to bulk up the frozen meal if you like. Even two packets of something like the Weight Watchers range of frozen meals will have less fat in them than a take-away, but you would still be doubling up on the rice or whatever carbohydrates are included, so try to avoid the second helping of carbs.

Even better you could *make* a curry or suitable alternative to your normal take-away. Add plenty of whatever spices are relevant to the dish as these are what will help to meet the need of your desire for a take-away – the chicken, beef, fish or pork in the dish isn't what it's about. It's all about the flavour of the sauce.

If you have got into the habit of also ordering prawn crackers or a side order then you need to think in advance about healthier alternatives if you don't think you could just leave them out. For example, try heating a few Broghies (look a little bit like prawn crackers and are just as crunchy, but very low in calories – I get these from Dunnes), or buy some very light crisps such as Treble Crunch or similar and put them in a bowl on the tray if that is what you would do with the prawn crackers.

If you tend to finish off your meal with something sweet, try a small, low-fat dessert, like a mini pot of mousse, or some pre-prepared stewed apple covered with some yogurt, or perhaps a few sweets you can suck. Any of these options will meet the need for something sweet without adding bucket-loads more fat.

If Sunday roasts are your thing then investigate how you can make them healthier. Focus on the meat and vegetables: roast the vegetables separately to the meat so they don't get drowned in fat – all they need is a drizzle/a few sprays of oil on a baking tray. Choosing lean meat (avoiding surrounding skin and fat no matter how crispy it is) and bulking up the vegetables will allow you to meet the craving for the ritual without sacrificing your weight loss. Unless the roasties are your Keepers do try to cut them down *a lot* for the moment. Baked spuds are a better way to go but even these should be cut back a lot. If you normally place pieces of bacon rasher over your chicken when roasting it, try turkey rashers as they are far less fattening and become just as crispy and tasty – just add them nearer the end of the cooking time for the chicken.

Is a bacon butty for your elevenses the thing you can't do without? If you can't cut it out, try grilling a rasher or two (turkey rasher would be even better) in the evening if you are tight on time and know you won't feel like it in the morning. You can then re-heat it in the microwave in the morning for breakfast, maybe with an egg (microwaveable to just the way you like it too). This should give you enough of the feeling of the butty without the heart attack and should tick the box long enough to last past your 11 a.m. trigger. Obviously not going to the place you buy the cardiac-arrest cake they call a breakfast roll is your best option, but if you have tried and failed on this one, then having the filling for breakfast as I have described will make it a whole lot easier for you to choose something healthier in the shop.

This kind of effort becomes *so* much easier when you have lost a bit of weight as then you have something you really want to protect.

Whenever you are making a healthier alternative make sure you give yourself a huge flavour kick. This is so important in order to feel satisfied and answer the desire for something tasty. So many people get an instant visual of insipid watery vegetables when they think of healthy eating so it is no wonder they begrudge giving up their favourite foods!

YOUR KEEPERS WILL KEEP YOU GOING!

Your Keepers will help you to stick with your eating plans and prevent that feeling of falling over the finish line at the weekend when most people struggle the most. Because you will not have denied yourself completely you won't have that 'to hell with this' moment when your good intentions go out the window.

Guideline No. 3: If You Stick It in Your Mouth, Stick It on the List – Keeping a Food Diary

When it comes to eating we all tend to have selective memory about what we consume. In fact, research has shown that even professional dieticians underestimate what they have eaten over the course of a day when they do not write it down. Keeping a food diary (pen and paper or digital) forces us to be accountable for everything we eat and is also a great way to see where patterns emerge to do with our eating. For example, we might notice that we eat well up until about 7 p.m. and suddenly the flood gates open and no food is safe. Or perhaps we tend to overeat only when we are alone or only when we are with a particular person. Identifying these patterns allows us to spend our food intake like a currency, spreading it evenly throughout the day/week, or cutting back in some areas so that we can 'spend it' in others.

I have to admit I found keeping a food diary a bit of a chore, but it did make me think twice before putting something in my mouth. It is a very similar effect to seeing ourselves in a mirror – becoming self-aware makes us behave better! One study showed that people who kept a food diary lost *twice* as much as their counterparts who didn't. Your diary should include columns for the date, food eaten, time and place of eating, the thought going through your mind (i.e. what is the voice in your head saying to you), the feeling(s) you have before eating, and the feeling(s) you experience after eating. I have given an example of what might be listed in each column in the sample diary below. Remember ALL your eating, not just the eating you regret, should be listed in your diary.

You might want to use a very small and portable notebook for your diary, or just have a specific piece of paper in your pocket or bag to serve as your diary each day. Just make sure to file them all together at the end of the week so that you can begin to see where patterns of eating and corresponding thoughts and feelings occur.

Date	Time & Place	Food Eaten	Thought	Feeling e.g. stress, anger, sadness, exhaustion, excitement, happiness, frustration	Feeling after Eating
12/1/13	12.05 in car	Sausage roll	I won't get a chance for lunch later – need energy	Frustration – know I'm just making excuse 'cos I want it	Fed up, angry with myself, fat, unhealthy

Make sure to keep your food diaries for a few months so that you can read back over them. Being reminded of how you felt after eating things you knew were not good for you is a brilliant motivating reminder to pause and think next time, before you stuff a piece of rubbish in your mouth. You may also be able to see times of day in your average week's schedule where your motivation crumbles, or that, for example, dealing with a specific person makes you reach for the chocolate. Food diaries provide the most personalised information you can get regarding your eating habits, what works for you and where the easy changes can be made. This knowledge will be your key to change.

WHAT ARE YOU DOING?

Decide how you will describe your new plans to yourself and others, but don't feel obliged to explain yourself to others if you don't want to.

The words you use to yourself and others will have quite an impact on how you feel about taking steps to improve your eating. 'Finding out what works for me' sounds a whole lot less arduous than 'I'm on a diet'.

Some other positive alternatives might be:

I'm making changes to my diet.
I'm tweaking my eating habits.
I'm changing my diet around a bit.
I'm gradually learning to eat better.
I'm losing the lard!

Guideline No. 4: Speeding Up Your Weight Loss – Exercise

Does your heart sink at the mention of exercise? If it does, hear this: exercise is not absolutely vital to weight loss, but it helps you to see results faster and that's a nice option to have. I hope that takes away some of the fear factor for you.

Weight loss is estimated to be approximately seventy per cent down to what you eat and thirty per cent down to your exercise routine for the average person. Of course, plenty of people stay slim without exercising and anyone who has ever stood on a treadmill knows just how much effort it takes to work off a very small number of calories, so if you can only focus your mind on one project for the moment, make it your food intake rather than exercise.

IT IS A FAR BETTER PLAN OF ACTION TO NOT EAT THE UNNECESSARY FOOD IN THE FIRST PLACE THAN TO THINK YOU WILL BE ABLE TO WORK IT OFF LATER. IF IT WERE THAT EASY TO WORK OFF THE LITTLE EXTRAS WE GIVE OURSELVES YOU WOULDN'T BE READING THIS BOOK.

Obviously, exercise is good for us in lots of ways, most particularly for the heart and lungs and also for our mental health. But one of the big benefits on offer to us with exercise is the opportunity to increase the amount of muscle mass we have in our body. Do this and we burn more calories, even asleep, than we do without the extra muscle. Muscle burns more calories than fat just to exist and that is a helpful thing to keep in mind if you are struggling to balance weight goals with your lifestyle.

I decided to take up jogging on the basis that I thought it would be a good calorie burner, would be something I could do whenever and wherever I had a few spare minutes and wouldn't involve driving anywhere, organising lockers or any other complications. I would never in a million years describe myself as a natural runner – I'm more of a plodder. And so I started plodding the streets where I live. Very, very slowly. My brother is a keen runner and he had heard the Olympic athlete Eamonn Coghlan say that the biggest mistake beginners make when starting to run is to start out too fast, instead of starting off slowly. This piece of advice was the most useful piece of information I ever got. It was the only thing that made me feel like giving jogging a go.

I had also read Gerry Duffy's wonderful book *Who Dares, Runs* about how he turned himself from an overweight smoker into an Ironman Decathlete.[4] It's a warm, honest, self-deprecating and inspirational read for anyone interested in taking up jogging. I highly recommend it. In the book Gerry talks about the times when pushing through exhaustion he just kept putting one foot in front of the other on the basis that this would eventually get him over the finish line. This was the attitude I adopted to get me started: don't even think about speed, just keep putting one foot in front of the other. Doing this spared me that awful feeling of breathlessness that brings any exercise to a grinding halt fairly quickly. At the outset I could probably have walked faster. But jogging was decidedly harder work. And then I just kept going, a little more and a little more, music blaring in my ears so that I couldn't hear my breathing (being able to hear myself breathe for some reason, always makes me feel instantly knackered).

In case you think I'm working towards some fabulous achievement in the running department, I'm not. I am still a plodder and probably always will be. In fact, after a few months of this plodding, people began to comment that they had seen me out. Kindly meant comments like, 'You're really into running now? That's great,' would make my heart sink, as I am fully aware of my slow progress in this department. 'Really into running' is probably not an accurate description of me. However, I have somewhat caught the shuffling/plodding/jogging bug and I do sometimes look forward to getting out. Mostly I do it because I think I should for my general health, and I try to just go before I think myself out of it. There have been days where I have been lapped by other runners (plenty of these) and days when I have lapped others, days when I felt delighted with myself and days when I couldn't do half of what I had done the day before. It doesn't matter. I get out and feel better for it afterwards. In fact, very early on in my plodding days I was feeling so chuffed with myself that I thought I would give one of those charity events a go.

WHEN CHARITY SHOULD HAVE STAYED AT HOME

I know many professional athletes use visualisation to increase the likelihood of them performing well on match day, but sometimes the big day doesn't quite work out as you had imagined it.

I had entered my first ever public charity walk/run in Dublin. It was promoted as a family friendly fun event in which you could choose to walk or run 5 or 10km. I wasn't sure that I could definitely jog 5km but thought I would put myself down for the 10km and could always walk the last 5km. Unfortunately all the beginner/fun runners seemed to stop at 5km so I found myself bringing up the rear of the field on the second half of the run. Everyone still going was at least jogging so I thought I had better struggle on. As the roads were closed off to traffic at many junctions I came across a few gardaí standing around their motorbikes. I sort of got used to them seeing me drag myself along, clearly not up to the job and got used to their few words of encouragement: 'nearly there ... keep going ... good on ya ...' etc. I tried to give a pathetic attempt at a smile back but was frankly too wrecked to make it happen.

Just as I entered the home stretch I heard a garda bike pulling up behind me. As he came alongside me I tried to muster enough of a polite smile in response to the words of encouragement I was expecting to hear. Instead he said, 'Sorry luv, but you'll have to move on to the pavement, we're reopening the roads.'

Dignity shattered!

For me jogging seemed the easiest exercise to try to fit into a busy life, but others may find that they prefer organised classes or going to a gym. When choosing an exercise to help you lose weight it is important to be honest with yourself about the intensity of the exercise. I really enjoy playing tennis, but my once-a-week game is nowhere near enough to help me lose weight. Similarly a once weekly round of golf might be great socially, but won't cut it for calorie burning. Walking, jogging, swimming, cycling and more high-intensity activities are likely to help you see results faster, and resistance training will help you build some muscle which makes your body burn more calories even while you sleep. Remember to avoid extremes of thinking when considering taking up or increasing your exercise regime. Beware of avoiding jogging 'because I'm no Sonia O'Sullivan' or avoiding swimming because you can't get to the pool three times a week. Just take it one week at a time, thinking about what you can fit in this week and what is practical for your weekdays and your weekends. Avoid mental expectations of yourself as a cyclist, runner, swimmer, etc., and just think about what you can do today that would help you burn some extra calories and give you that fantastic energised, virtuous and justifiably self-righteous glow.

7

MORE MORSELS TO REMEMBER

Chunking Your Ladder

How do you see the weight you need to lose? Do you think of it as one big piece of weight – like one and a half stone or X kilograms – the kind of thing you might ask for at the butcher's? Or perhaps in terms of 'I want to weigh Y'?

You may never have paid attention to how you think of the weight you want to lose, but doing so will really help to make your weight-loss goals more achievable. 'Chunking' is a term used in psychology to describe the process of breaking down a big task into smaller, more manageable parts. If you have a lot of weight to lose then it can seem a bit of a mountain to climb, which only strengthens the desire to put it off until you are 'in the mood', 'in the zone', etc.

Set aside some time to draw up a weight ladder or podium – the weight-loss equivalent of a time line – to mentally break down the total amount of weight you want to lose into smaller blocks. Identify target weights along the way where you can have a little solo party in your bathroom or just in your head once achieved … think 'Cha cha cha!' or 'And he's done it again. This man is unstoppable!' etc.

Write your starting weight at the top of the ladder and then draw a line downwards. The points on the weight ladder do not need to be evenly spaced, decreasing in even half stones for example. The first point on your podium should be the lowest point of your starting weight allowing for your body's natural fluctuations.

Your next step on the weight ladder could be perhaps an even X stone or a round number of kilograms or an even X stone seven pounds or a number of kilos divisible by five. The next might be another three pounds or two kilos under the next round number. Going into a new weight bracket, such as going from eleven stone something to ten stone thirteen or from seventy-something to sixty-nine kilos is a cause for celebration. Another step on the podium might be losing five or ten per cent of your body weight, or getting to exactly one or two stone/five or ten kilos above your target weight and another an even ten pounds above it, etc. It really doesn't matter how you chunk it as long as each step has some meaning to you.

A fun 3D alternative to this is to actually build the podium, perhaps on a bathroom window sill, using pound packs of lard as building blocks and any little figurine you choose to represent you gradually moving up towards the top spot on the podium. At the very least it will put a smile on your face in the morning and blocks of lard are a brilliant way to make you appreciate what you have achieved each time you lose a pound of weight. One word of warning: don't put them anywhere the sun comes through – you don't want your weight-loss podium becoming your new flooring!

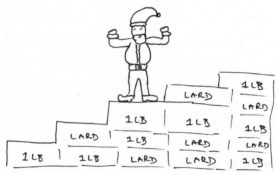

SANTA QUITE ENJOYED HIS NEW JOB ON THE
PODIUM NOW THAT HIS BUSY SEASON WAS OVER

To Recap …

You need to give yourself the best chance of getting past the lowest point of your normal weight fluctuations in order to really feel you are making progress. In order to achieve this you need to:

1 **Be honest about your Keepers** – have you really reduced or swapped for an alternative that is A LOT lower in fat and calories? Also beware of 'Keeper Creep'; when things are going well it is easy to become overly relaxed about the portion size of your Keeper(s) – they are not supposed to be a licence to pig out!

2 **Cut those carbs** – the amount you will need depends on your levels of activity during your average day. However, if you are overweight you are probably eating too many of them. True, running around after a young child or out and about on appointments does burn calories without you even realising it, but again, if you are reading this book your excess calories aren't shifting. Cut down carbohydrates *a lot* and remember that your Keepers are very likely to count towards your carb intake for the day. As we have said, we are all kidding ourselves but not our bodies when we use the food pyramid as our excuse for eating carbs. Just remember the carbs section of the pyramid has the widest girth!

NUTS ABOUT NUTS?

I would also caution against snacking on nuts as many health books recommend. People who are overweight have not learned or have forgotten when enough is enough. Nuts are full of nutrients but also fat, so either leave them out for the moment or ask a professional for advice on how many you should be eating, taking into account what you are already eating, including your Keepers. It would be preferable to reintroduce nuts into your diet when you have weaned yourself off your Keepers. Nutritionists might argue that when you get all the good fats from nuts you won't crave the bad stuff, like your Keepers. This argument presumes that you listen to your body's signals for what it needs. But when was the last time you were in tune with your body's needs? People who are overweight respond to emotional (I'm stressed/bored) and situational (in the car/ at the desk) cues to trigger their eating, so the perfect balance of good fats is something to aim for but probably won't get a look in for the foreseeable future.

3   **Tweak what you eat – pluck your low-hanging fruit** – change your sauces, grill don't fry, 'interest-up' salads and vegetables and get kids' rubbish out of the house or at the very least out of sight. If they are not there you can't eat them and they won't suggest themselves to you.

4   **Be prepared** – in the car, work or kitchen have the good stuff easily to hand. People who overeat have developed a habit of just sticking something in their mouths – for the time being make sure it's an apple or other fruit, a few raisins if you like them, a piece of sugar-free gum, or a sucky sweet if really necessary. Once you have lost a good deal of weight you will be far more motivated and feel energised enough to introduce and maintain healthier snacking habits long term with ease. Again you need to keep in mind that habits are deeply entrenched in us and we need to create new habits by repetition and reward – in this case feeling great. Getting rid of the 'stick-something-in-my-mouth' (even something healthy) habit is a medium- to long-term project. But by lessening the reward of eating by changing to eating something less sweet or fatty, you weaken the old habit making it easier to dissolve completely later on.

Similarly, if you know you are going to have a big night out eat something light but filling during the day, such as home-made soup. Get real here. Don't decide that you are going to eat as if it was a normal day if you know you are going out in the evening for a meal. It really is not that difficult to down two days' worth of calories in a night between alcohol, nibbles, dinner, desserts, cheeses, and even possibly chips on the way home. And no, you probably won't work it all off on the dance floor so stop kidding yourself.

Mental Maths

People who are overweight are terrible at maths and brilliant at fooling themselves. Watch what you eat in passing and watch what you tell yourself. It is quite possible for someone to 'inhale' a packet of crisps at the bar while waiting for their pint to be poured and chatting to someone so they probably don't even remember doing it. And it is, as I have already talked about, actually quite difficult to work off excess calories taken in and, therefore, a far better idea to make a little extra effort not to eat them in the first place. It is so easy to make a quick mental tot in your head as you order a Danish pastry with your coffee:

I'm going for a walk this evening with a friend so I'll walk it off then.

OR

> *I'm coaching the kids at soccer on Saturday. I'll work it off then.*

In both cases the person probably has no idea of the calorie and fat content of the Danish or exactly how many calories their walk or coaching session will burn, so cannot possibly know if they will burn it off. In addition, unless they record it in a diary they are very likely to forget it and will use exactly the same walk/ coaching session to justify the extra helping of dinner they have that evening. This is also why diarying everything you eat is so important.

We are absolutely brilliant at rationalising things to ourselves. If you find yourself making any such mental arithmetic around food, presume that it is all lies and that you are, in fact, completely wrong. Eat whatever it is and you will put on weight. This is probably what you have been doing for years. Your maths has never been good in the food department.

Lieing Eyes

The visual image and beliefs that we hold about certain foods have a massive impact on our eating and our girths. Do you see all sandwiches as equal?

Do you think this staple Irish lunch is nutritionally balanced because it contains carbohydrate (bread), protein (meat filling) perhaps some calcium rich dairy produce (cheese), and some salad? Do you ever ask yourself if you have had enough carbohydrate already today? If the meat filling is lean? How many calories come with the calcium and anyway do you need more calcium? Is butter or a calorie-laden mayonnaise used in the mix?

Do you see tuna mayonnaise as healthy because it's fish? Or coleslaw, because it's salad? Have you ever thought about the fat content of the mayonnaise these supposedly 'healthy' foods are floating in? What about Caesar salad? Do you presume it's healthy because it has got the word salad in its title? The average fat content of a Caesar salad is massive. Swap it for a different dressing.

How about take-aways? You probably know they're bad for you, but how much do you really deeply *know* this? Sometime when you get a chance carry out this exercise. Have a look online to find out the fat content of your chosen take-away meal. Buy a block of lard or goose fat and weigh out the equivalent amount. Wrap it in cellophane and leave it in the fridge or somewhere you will see it regularly. This is what you are swallowing each time you eat a take-away. The fat has just melted. You could go one step further and microwave the fat or put it in a saucepan over the heat to liquify it. This will give you an even more realistic image of what you are putting in your mouth. In fact, you could do this exercise with absolutely any food you know you shouldn't eat or want to eat less of. Positive affirmations are all very well, but sometimes a good dose of realism will work wonders.

Many of the mental pictures we have of food are unconscious and automatic. You may have made these assumptions ten or even fifty years ago and never questioned them since. In fact, even at the outset you may not have made them consciously but inherited them from a parent or other family member. It is only by becoming aware of them that you can begin to get the more logical part of your brain to assess whether or not these are accurate and useful assumptions or whether, as with the take-away, you need to get real.

Attentional Bias

When we are overweight we have selective attention and seek out information related to food and exercise that is in keeping with what we already believe. In psychology this is referred to as Attentional Bias.

Our minds do everything they can to maintain our beliefs, and much more readily see evidence that supports our existing beliefs and ignore or honestly don't notice evidence to the contrary. So when we have a coffee or lunch with a slim friend we see them having a large portion of carbs or something sweet, we do that pathetically bad mental arithmetic about burning it off later and make unconscious and wrong assumptions about what our slim friend will also eat later in the day. However, our slim friend will make adjustments in their diet for the rest of the day to allow for what they have eaten earlier. They will either do this unconsciously by not eating again until they are hungry or consciously by eating something lighter for the remainder of the day. Don't waste your time on excuses about life being unfair. Except for a small minority of people who have truly fast metabolisms all their lives, life is not more unfair to you than anyone else in the eating world. If you are overweight you probably just eat more. Face it. If you do have a naturally thin friend then get over it. Moaning about it won't help you to lose weight. Accept it and focus on your own plan of action:

- Your Keepers

- Your swapping and tweaking
- Your food diary
- Your exercise

If all the kick-ass, all-or-nothing style diets haven't worked for you, you are I hope now beginning to understand why. You were swimming against the tide of biology, the way your brain is wired. Continuing this disgraceful display of mixed metaphors, what you are going to do now is negotiate with your unconscious mind, beg or just plain sneak your changes past when it's not paying attention. As we have said before, to do this you need to make small changes first, following the path of least resistance, picking off the low-hanging fruit, without upsetting the apple cart.

The Pyramid of Change

Making these changes and losing weight as fast as is healthily possible will allow your unconscious mind to register the benefits of change and to gradually lay down new neural pathways for new eating habits. So, in true stepping up to the plate mode you need to set out a hierarchy of changes to be made, in increasing levels of difficulty.

To some extent this is what the Fabulous Jelly

programme is doing for you anyway. A step-by-step approach to change is inherent in the programme. You begin by identifying your low-hanging fruit and make swaps and tweaks rather than giving up anything. Making a pyramid of change is another way of 'chunking' the tasks needed for weight loss. Instead of looking at losing weight as a general all round pain, your pyramid will allow you to see which parts could be described as 'really not that bad', which might feel at this moment like a fate worse than death, and which lie somewhere in the middle.

For example, when you sit down to think about it, you might decide that you could easily enough stop having biscuits in the office with your coffee as lots of people just have a diet yogurt. This might go at the bottom of your pyramid – at entry level. Perhaps you think you could just about manage to have coffee but not cake when meeting friends or business colleagues? This could go in the mid section of the pyramid. Maybe you think that snacks on the couch in front of the TV are going to be your nemesis? This will go at or near the top of your pyramid.

Put as many levels as you like into your pyramid. In fact, the more you put in the better as it means you are breaking down the challenge of weight loss into smaller and smaller parts, some of which won't seem particularly difficult when viewed in this way. It is likely that you will need to keep adding to your pyramid at the start of the Fabulous Jelly programme as you will begin to pay much more attention to when and where you eat.

Note that in the example given overleaf one of the levels is actually an emotional trigger (anger) rather than a particular time of day.

What Next for Your Pyramid?

After you have drawn up your pyramid then you need to put an action for now or later beside each level. Your plan of action involves starting at the point of least resistance. This is the low-hanging fruit. For example, changes like swapping to a low-fat version of a product. Or looking up (if not yet making) a few new quick recipe ideas for busy evenings. Or buying the freezer foils you never got around to buying so you can freeze dinner portions and be prepared for the times you arrive home hungry. Or even buying some frozen low-fat meals to begin with. Or if a muffin with your coffee is your Keeper then how about going to a coffee shop that displays the fat and calorie content of their products online or in store.

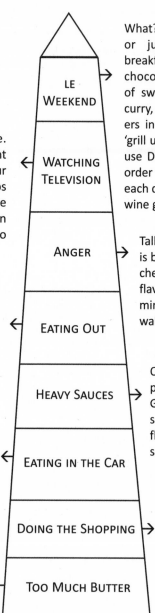

LE WEEKEND

What? The whole weekend or just evenings/Sunday breakfast? Try a light hot chocolate drink instead of sweets, cook your own curry, buy in turkey rashers in advance and have a 'grill up' instead of a fry up, use Diet 7-Up for spritzers, order sparkling water with each drink and ask for it in a wine glass.

WATCHING TELEVISION

Prepare in advance. Sometimes we just want to stick something in our mouths. Try fruit kebabs on skewers, a water ice pop, broghie, or even once see how it feels to not eat.

ANGER

Talking to a trusted friend is best for this. If need to chew, chew gum – fruit flavoured if don't feel like mint. Get air if you can, walk or march.

EATING OUT

Have some light, salty nibbles before you go, ditch the carbs – they aren't the bit with the flavour. Bring a boiled sweet to have as dessert.

HEAVY SAUCES

On what? Probably a pile of tasteless carbs. Go for tomato-based sauces on veg.: stronger flavours are more satisfying.

EATING IN THE CAR

Always have wipes and a small bin bag in the car. Use fruit, gum, boiled sweets, mints etc.

DOING THE SHOPPING

Plan ahead. Do you need to buy your Keepers? Have these to look forward to when you get home.

TOO MUCH BUTTER

You will be cutting carbs anyway, which will help. Try various alternative spreads.

Although the Fabulous Jelly programme does not count calories, it does make you aware of calories, so finding out the calorie and fat content of your muffin and comparing it to the recommended daily calorie intake for men and women, less some for weight loss, will give you an idea of what percentage of your daily allowance you are swallowing with each bite. In general, muffins are not a good idea for your Keepers unless you make a low-calorie, low-fat variety at home.

If coming home and stuffing your face before you've taken your coat off is on your list, your plan of action might be to have bottled sparkling water easily to hand, as this might be enough to satisfy the urge to just have something (this one works really well for me). Or you might have a bag of chopped carrots to stick into some hummus in the fridge, or fruit that you actually like – maybe kiwi or a pineapple already peeled and cored. As soon as you have begun to lose weight this kind of response to triggers becomes so much easier, because now you have something worth protecting. The important thing at the beginning is to make your action plans *realistic for you*. So often diet books tell people to avoid snacking by going for a walk or having a relaxing bath. This is complete rubbish for the majority of people for most of their day. How easy is it when minding children to simply disappear out for a walk? And suggesting people have a bath at work is just silly – can you imagine the queue at the door? Find realistic alternatives and swaps. You should find that just being allowed your Keepers is enough to get you through these moments and that you are willing to eat the peach rather than the pie when you have your treat to look forward to later in the day, tomorrow or later in the week.

Cooking

You can lose weight without changing how much you cook on the Fabulous Jelly programme. It is designed to demand as little change as possible of you. However, in the longer term, life will be much more interesting and enjoyable if you learn to cook or cook differently. But even this change should be done gradually. Most of us have had one of those phases where we swallow an entire recipe book and buy a shop full of herbs and spices that we use once and end up throwing out a year later. Aim to try out a maximum of one or two new recipes a week that really appeal to you and/or that you think might be suitable for all the family. If you are not the one who does the cooking in your household take some time to decide on a *realistic for you* strategy for dealing with this issue. For some it might be very easy: the person who cooks may be delighted to try out some new recipes and pleased that you are taking an interest. As a wife and mother I can guarantee you that thinking of something for the family to eat every evening can be a real grind. Your partner may feel the same way. So perhaps you could agree to do the cooking one evening a week even if they suggest the dish. Or swap it around and you agree to look up an idea for something tasty, they cook and you promise at the very least to stay with them, watch, learn and generally keep them company. The recipes don't have to involve lots of ingredients – keep things simple. It might mean just grilling some fish sprinkled with a few herbs and maybe roasting some vegetables that you know you like. If you don't like it when you try it, forget it. Healthy recipes aren't about 'being good'. We already know such resolutions don't work. In any cookery book you choose you are likely to use only a very small percentage of the recipes featured and this is true of readers whether or not they are aiming to lose weight. In fact, according to a recent UK survey, over half the cookbooks bought as Christmas presents go unread because people are put off by complicated recipes and expensive ingredients. The research showed that the average British adult owns ten cookbooks and has only ever used four of them. Sometimes it's nice to know we are average! Browsing recipes online might be your best bet.

Coffee and Small Pleasures

Beware of liquid calories and/or fat in things like fruit juices and especially coffee. Again, our tendency to forget about these calories is based on how we visualise them. Remember the Picture Superiority Effect we talked about in Chapter 2? Liquid doesn't look like it could be full of fat because it doesn't have that solid heavy look. It's because the power of how we visualise things affects our behaviour that the Irish government introduced graphic pictures of smoking-related diseases on cigarette packs. A picture is worth a thousand words as they say.

Look for better alternatives to your regular coffee if it is heavy on the calories. Cream on top, etc., is just making your weight-loss goal further away unless it just has to be your Keeper. Could you switch from a latte to an Americano with a good bit of frothed skimmed milk in it? As so much of your coffee experience is sensory you may be surprised to find that switching to a smaller size is easier than you expected as a smaller size still provides the taste, smell, heat and perhaps opportunity for a chat that you get from your regular size. Stay clear of energy drinks too. Remember that scientists measure energy in calories – that's what calories are! Would you drink it if it was called a 'calorie drink'?

8

CONTROL BRIEFS

How much do you think you are responsible for your weight gain? How much do you think losing weight is up to you and how much to luck, genetics, etc.? If you were able to relate to some or all of the examples of all-or-nothing thinking in Chapter 4 you may well be unconsciously disempowering yourself. Below are a few more examples of things overweight people believe and tell themselves.

Have you muttered anything along the lines of ...

My family are all big – it's in our genes.

I put on weight easily.

I just have to look at a cake to put on the weight.

My spouse keeps buying goodies for the kids – it's impossible to live in our home and lose weight.

I've no willpower.

It is how it is.

It's just me.

It's the luck of the draw.

It's all down to the roll of the dice.

All of these comments smack of what is known as an 'external locus of control'. Locus of control, a term first created by a guy called Julian Rotter (b. 1916) is a psychological concept relating to where you see control as being located – within you or external to you. Each of us develops a locus of control, largely unconsciously, by the way our parents and important adults in our lives behaved. For example, were you encouraged to make age appropriate decisions for yourself or were you still being told to change your underwear at the age of fifteen? If you wanted to wear a particular outfit to a party were you encouraged to make sure it was clean and ready for the event or was it still being washed and laid out for you when you were twenty? Did you see a parent take control of situations or would you say they often gave up? For example, if they were hard done by on an issue at work did they make an appointment to speak to the boss the next day or did they just not bother turning up for work or have a drink and get angry? Did you often hear the phrase 'that's life' bandied about? Of course, not all situations are controllable and sometimes all that a person can do is to try to 'chip away' at whatever part of the problem they do have control over. But again, becoming aware of how we view the world gives us the chance to ask ourselves if these views are helpful to us or are hindering us. Sometimes these views aren't just learned from parents but are also picked up from the culture of the country you grew up in. The point is, do you see control as being within you or external to you – in the lap of the gods as it were? If you think you have little or no control over your weight then you are very unlikely to get up off your behind and do something about it. You'll just take it bravely on one of your chins.

The problem with all of the above statements is that they are so deeply entrenched in our unconscious that we either never think about them at all or we say them as if they are fact. Set in stone. Not modifiable in any way. And, of course, very few friends or family are going to be rude enough to actually challenge them for fear of putting the blame squarely on your shoulders. And so they nod and lament with you, perhaps co-conspirators in the game because if they have weight to lose too then it makes them feel better if you believe the same tat. Maybe you share a joke together about the skinny and miserable brigade and then you tuck into whatever it is that got you into this mess in the first place.

Beware of 'Learned Helplessness'

Learned helplessness is a psychological concept, first identified by Martin Seligman in 1967. It occurs when people or animals learn or mis-learn that they have no control over unwanted outcomes or events. When this happens the animal or person stops making any attempts to change events but instead passively accepts things as they are, no matter how unwanted or unpleasant. This can be very relevant to weight loss.

Previous failed diet strategies affect people in different ways depending on what they attribute the failure to. For example, when two people fall off the diet wagon one might comment, 'That diet is ridiculous. It doesn't allow any sort of social life,' while another might say, 'I've never had any willpower. I can never stick to anything.'

It's fairly obvious that the first person attributes their failure to the inflexibility of the diet plan and will be motivated to choose more carefully next time. But there probably will be a next time. On the other hand, the second person attributes their failure to their own weakness, which, just to make things worse, they generalise to an all-pervading weakness as opposed to just relevant to the failed diet. This person is a whole lot less likely to try again or will fail before they even begin another diet because they have 'learned' that they have no control over the outcome.

In schools, children who believe all outcomes (such as grades achieved) are a result of their general ability fare much worse than children who believe that results are down to how much they have learned so far (mastery-oriented). If a child views poor grades as being down to poor ability they will tend to give up much quicker than those who believe that they just haven't yet learned enough or were not motivated enough at exam time. Poor ability seems insurmountable to the child, lack of mastery is temporary.

It's not that there is necessarily absolutely no truth in some of the statements, it's just that taking them on board as a sort of universal truth means that we never question them or tease them apart a bit – just like the beliefs we spoke about earlier. You need to question where you think control over your weight is.

In unashamedly cheesy terms:

IN YOUR LIFE, ARE YOU HOLDING THE REINS OR HOLDING ON TO THE SADDLE (FOR DEAR LIFE)?

'Ah', you say, 'all this positive self-talk is all very well but in the real world the hand you have been dealt does matter. Real life isn't fair.'

My answer is you're right, real life isn't fair. GET OVER IT. Find your own phrase that says 'Oh well' and work with what you have.

Yes you may well have a friend who can eat everything that stays still long enough to be eaten and remains slim. This is completely irrelevant to you. Deal with the facts you are faced with and don't waste time moaning. At the end of your moan you will still be overweight and they will still be slim.

BRINGING THE LOCUS OF CONTROL INWARDS: FIND YOURSELF SOME RELEVANT ROLE MODELS OF THE WEIGHT-LOSS WORLD THAT SHARE THE SAME STRUGGLES AS YOU.

Get yourself some role models to inspire you. Don't bother with airbrushed photos in fashion magazines. Go online or buy weight-loss magazines and save newspaper articles that give real life stories of people who have lost weight. Print/tear them out and put them somewhere you can see them regularly – like beside the sink where you brush your teeth, or on the side of the fridge. We tend to believe people that we see as being similar to us in some way more than people that are very different. Sometimes these similarities are imagined, sometimes not.

Before and after photos are great visual fodder for your brain. Highlight any tips or advice they give as to how they dealt with temptation or difficult times and what they found most helpful.

Addressing Some of Your Learned Helplessness

My family are all big – it's in our genes.

Yes if your mother was overweight when she gave birth to you, you may have inherited a tendency to put on weight. This is like a chronic disease that means you need to take *more* care of your diet than others. Again, it's down to how we visualise things. Because a tendency to obesity isn't something that we initially need medical appointments or daily medication for, we tend to think of it as more of a vanity issue, like you might have preferred to be born with black hair instead of brown, or wanted to be taller, etc. It's not. If you truly have a tendency to obesity you are living with a chronic disease and need to take action.

Bringing the locus of control inwards: You have already done some work in this book to identify what has worked for you in the past and what hasn't. By the time you have finished reading this book you will also know just how many 'pieces' of you cause weight gain, e.g. your tendency to all-or-nothing thinking, your sense of locus of control, your negative thinking habits, etc. You need to find a person or a programme that works on all of these pieces, to create an eating programme that considers both these unconscious factors and your goals.

I put on weight easily.

Yes, but probably only because you have a big appetite. You may even have stretched your stomach and forgotten how to recognise the chemical message for fullness that your brain sends you. You need to do something about both.

Bringing the locus of control inwards: You have tried but it's hard. Yes, it can be. But you were probably working against how your mind works in the past. The whole point of the Fabulous Jelly programme is to learn about what's going on in your brain around the issue of eating so that you can learn to work with, not against, it. As you have already seen, there's a lot in there. That's why you are going to follow the programme to lose weight as quickly and as painlessly as is healthily possible so that you are not working against all your body's natural instincts.

I have no willpower.

None? Do you get out of bed in the morning? Do you get yourself to work on time, hold down a job or normally manage to keep your cool with your children? You have willpower. But you need to understand how it works and why and when it seems to abandon you.

Bringing the locus of control inwards: At this stage you are perhaps beginning to realise that there are loads of things going on in your head that you are not consciously aware of, things you don't choose to think and feelings you don't choose to feel. Most of us go through our lives without ever taking the time to learn about how our minds work and to what extent we can choose what and how we think. But doing so has a huge impact on how we feel and how we behave and what we achieve in life, such as healthy relationships, rewarding work, etc. This is what is known as the Cognitive Triad – the interlinking of our thoughts (cognitions), our emotions (affect) and behaviour. Willpower, or 'self-regulation' as it is known in psychological research, is one area well worth taking a look at.

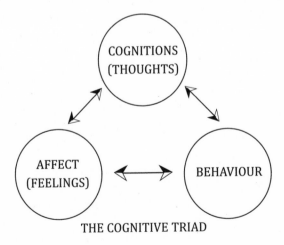

THE COGNITIVE TRIAD

Should you go down River Nile today you're in for a big surprise.

Should you go down River Nile today you'd better go in a smaller size ...

Some people's mothers warn their children to always wear clean underwear in case they are knocked down by a car and have to be brought to hospital. But no one could have foreseen this ...

I remember a romantic three-day boat trip down the Nile with my husband some years ago. We were having a ball. Each day we were taken by a guide to visit some of the endless number of fabulous sites and ruins that make Egypt one of those places you have just got to see in your lifetime. I adore all that stuff and was in my element.

Of course, back on board it was another day at the 'office' for the male staff who were running the boat. They did the usual sort of stuff, like manning the enquiry desk, catering, cleaning, organising evening entertainment – and knicker art. Yes, I kid you not, knicker art.

After a morning's tour we came back to find all our underwear laid out on the bed in the shape of two smiley faces, one dark, the other blonde. It was actually really brilliant. A colourful chain of socks, knickers, bras, swimwear and underpants had been skilfully twisted and shaped into two very good impressions of us both. But if only someone had warned me! I would have had only the loveliest and smallest of artistic options casually placed in the drawers for the artists – perfect for doing chiselled chins and much higher cheekbones than they gave me!

You have been warned. Could your under-garments be mistaken for the bedspread? Don't wait until you are at goal weight to make sure you feel good about how you look. Treating yourself to some small, low-cost outfits (or pretty underwear) will really help to keep up your motivation and replenish your willpower.

Mental self-talk can chatter on in the backgrounds of our minds for a lifetime. By bringing it to the forefront of our minds we can tease apart fact from fiction and useful from just plain mean. If you feel flattened or defeated in your attempts to lose weight you may have relatively recently (mis-)learned that you don't have what it takes to get to your goal weight. Having read through some of the examples above, you should now be more able to notice where you place control of your weight-loss goals and to have the confidence to challenge these beliefs where necessary.

9

'YOU WILL, YOU WILL, YOU WILL ...'

Willpower is a topic that has only relatively recently come back into favour with psychologists. For many years willpower was seen as a throwback to the austerity years of wartime Europe. It was equated with an old-fashioned sense of duty and many psychologists even stated that willpower does not exist. As people began to rebuild their lives after the Second World War, commerce grew, the population had more spending power and the power of advertising grew. Psychological research in the 1970s showed that people with higher self-confidence seemed to do better and be happier in life, and so began a whole pop psychology culture advising us all to love ourselves, value ourselves and generally think we were the kingpin. All good to some extent until 'Tiger Mom' spoiled the party.

Researchers measuring the effects of the feel-good era noticed that although children raised with lots of positive self-worth and praise were indeed highly confident in their abilities, their actual performance was lower than their Eastern counterparts raised on a much stricter regime. High self-confidence did not equate to good performance. More recently books like *Battle Hymn of the Tiger Mother* hit the headlines chiefly because the author, Amy Chua, told us what we probably already knew in our heart of hearts but couldn't quite handle: in comparison to the East, Western societies were turning out spoiled children who couldn't handle a difficult turnip.[5]

Our young people were having every problem in the school-yard fixed for them, every battle fought for them and a sense of achievement given to them for free. They appeared to have no need to strive for anything, to work or save for anything, and never to have to deal with disappointment and straightforward failure. Even more recently, in Ireland the Celtic Tiger cubs grew up on shopping as a Saturday afternoon pastime and eating in restaurants as a weekly event. As the country enjoyed a 'live-for-today' philosophy, long-term savings plans went by the wayside and luxury items became the norm.

As a friend once said of her much younger sister:

She'd buy her bread and milk in Brown Thomas if she could!

But things have changed and now there is a new raft of research on willpower – how we get it, use it and lose it. For a brilliant read on the subject of willpower take a look at Baumeister and Tierney's book, *Willpower. Rediscovering the Greatest Human Strength.*[6]

Contrary to beliefs held previously in the psychology world, willpower most certainly does exist. However, as any chronic dieter can testify, it varies from person to person. We can blame genetics for some of this difference, but the variation between people is mostly down to upbringing and how we use willpower in our daily lives.

Willpower is like a muscle – if we use it, it gets stronger. If you were brought up with a high value on achievement then you are more likely to have a sense that achieving your chosen goal, be it health, wealth, happiness or something else, is up to you (internal locus of control). You may have been pushed by your parents to study or to stick at a course or hobby that you wanted to run like hell from. Perhaps your parents told you they would match whatever you managed to save up from your pocket money over a month to help you buy a more expensive toy, rather than making an immediate purchase of something small the moment you got the money into your hands. If this was you, you are more likely to be the person who can in adulthood fight the temptation to take a coffee break until after a document is written or a difficult phone call is made. You can thank your parents for helping you to strengthen your willpower muscle. But if this is not you, don't think you are off the hook!

It is never too late to start working on your willpower, but like every other mental event we have spoken about, learn how it works first.

Budget Your Willpower

The ability to control our thoughts, feelings or behaviour requires mental energy. By this I don't mean some metaphorical spirit or essence. I mean glucose from the body – and a lot of it. Your brain takes up about two per cent of your body weight but uses up roughly twenty per cent of your energy (calorie) intake. Within this twenty per cent some of this is used to keep the unconscious processes ticking over, but most is used up with things that require mental effort in our daily lives. It's like revving up the engine of a car – it guzzles fuel. There are SO many events in our day that take their toll on your mental energy: the guilt you experience as you hit the snooze button one time too many, the effort required to get up out of bed, the remembering of everything you need to do in the day, the self-control not to blast the car horn when another driver cuts across you, the effort required to keep your mouth shut when someone annoys you or you need to keep a confidence, the self-control needed to not have a quick peek at your Facebook page during work, the nagging feeling that you know you need to contact someone you don't want to talk to though the feeling won't go away until you do, the decision at the super-market about what the family will eat for dinner, the motivation to get up off the couch and go for a walk, to keep going when you're tired, etc. There are thousands upon thousands of mini decisions and events that deplete our mental energy, our brain glucose and our willpower. Whether we are resisting buying something, saying something or trying to do something, our brain takes the energy from the same reserve.

So apart from willpower being like a muscle that needs to be worked so as to improve its strength, it is also like a currency that we spend. Use it and it runs out. To use a different metaphor, on the one hand practising using self-control pumps water into the reservoir, but at the other end, if we let the water flow freely out, the reservoir is likely to run dry. In their book Baumeister and Tierney report on a marriage guidance counsellor who advised his clients to return home from work earlier than they were because their reserves of self-control were being 'spent' at work. This resulted in them struggling and failing to remain polite and patient with their partner. They begin to experience what is known as 'decision fatigue' – the inability to make any more choices that require a clear mind and the self-control to bite their tongue, resist saying something and look after their relationship. It turns out that the old adage about keeping your best manners for home seems even more necessary in our stressful modern lives.

The fact that willpower needs glucose is not good news for anyone hoping to rely on it for losing weight. It means that just when you are feeling peckish and in need of a good munch, i.e. when your blood glucose is low, your willpower is also low. This is why so many dieters report that they can control their food intake without problem during the day but in the evenings their willpower deserts them. In fact, even people who generally score high on tests of self-control only do marginally better at using self-control for eating than those who are 'self-control' challenged. (There is justice in the world after all!) It is likely that the people who exhibit self-control in their daily lives probably use some very clear-cut rules for themselves such as on Thursdays I will play football (even if I don't feel like it), or I take a coffee break at 11.15 a.m., Monday to Friday. However, as we cannot give up eating, such clear-cut strategies are more difficult to apply in the weight-loss world.

When researchers used scans to look at what happens in the brain when a person exerts self-control they identified activity in a part of the brain known as the Dorsolateral Prefrontal Cortex (DLPFC).[7] When our willpower is spent, activity in the DLPFC decreases. Although many of us would consider ourselves experts in the 'Oh sod it, I'll have ...' moments, psychologists looked for slightly more scientific external signals of this breakdown in self-control. In fact, it was some of Baumeister's own research that showed that when our willpower is at its lowest ebb we experience all emotions with greater intensity, so that, for example, a sad film will have us drowning the sitting room with tears, a small bang will feel like a run in with a sledgehammer and surprisingly happy things will have us bouncing off the ceilings. Every emotion, good and bad, seems to be intensified.[8] Unfortunately this includes cravings. You crave the sugary snack because your brain needs glucose to give you willpower, but you need willpower to avoid the sugary snack.

Relying *solely* on willpower to keep you in control on any weight-loss programme is a waste of time. In fact, you probably knew this already from experience, but so keen are we all on becoming better and brighter versions of ourselves that we just won't learn from previous mistakes. Instead we fill ourselves with false hopes in every new eating plan that comes our way, without any regard for our starting point, our lifestyles or our previous histories. Hope and a focus on the future keep us happy and healthy. But hope also sells and false hope delays us in getting to where we want to go. Get real and get going.

EXTREMES DO NOT WORK!

GIVING UP FOOD YOU LOVE DOESN'T WORK!

YOU HAVE BEEN WARNED!

Of course, we all want the quick fix, because in today's world we are constantly bombarded with things competing for our attention, which has resulted in us having shorter attention spans than previous generations and in a demand for more of everything, faster. But remember that asking the body to deny itself food that is necessary for its very survival is what we appropriately called 'One great humdinger of an ask'. The body simply won't let you. Trying to push our bodies to resist things it has learned are full of glucose (sugar) and, therefore, beneficial to survival, is going to set off alarm bells regarding our very existence. You will awaken the wrong giant within – the ever-powerful, unconscious, instinctive mind. The one that keeps our heart beating, our blood flowing, our immune cells fighting infection, our lungs working, our eyelids fluttering and our noses sniffing out the pheromones of a potential mate. There is an obvious link between all of these tasks. These activities of the unconscious brain support our very existence … and you think it's a good idea to take it on? To deny the unconscious some type of food forever or restrict food intake so much the body thinks there is a famine? Are you feeling lucky? Your unconscious mind, where your body's survival instinct resides, will wipe the proverbial floor with you

– as you have probably already seen when it slows your metabolism just when you thought you were doing so well on the latest crash diet.

Don't try to blast your way to a healthier weight with willpower and restriction. All the science shows it won't work – at least not for long. This is why the Fabulous Jelly programme takes a gentler and more sustainable approach. Nothing too drastic that would ring any survival instinct alarm bells, just a gentle eye-level-and-below spring clean of your main weight-gain culprits, such as too many carbs and heavy sauces, and of course identifying your Keepers. No trying to suddenly dump habits built up over a lifetime. As we have seen from the research, we only have one 'reservoir' of willpower, so we need to apply ourselves to one challenge at a time to give ourselves any chance of success. That's why we have our Keepers. The little home comforts we can't do without just yet. As we make changes to our general diet we will gradually change our tastes for those too. But not yet.

10

CRAVINGS AND OTHER CRITTERS

Surveys have shown that nearly one hundred per cent of women and seventy per cent of men experience food cravings, so they need no introduction.[9] In fact, they are firmly on the map along with craving drugs or lovely shoes – they stimulate the same emotion, memory and reward areas of the brain. For many years researchers have argued against the existence of food addiction, no matter how many of us may classify ourselves as chocoholics. But in some interesting research the National Institute on Drug Abuse in the US has scanned the brains of obese people and shown that they look just like the brains of drug addicts in the areas of the brain relating to pleasure and self-control.[10] They also showed that, just like those of drug addicts, the brains of obese people react increasingly strongly to seeing anything the person associates with getting their food 'fix', such as seeing the food itself or the packaging etc., but the reaction to actually eating the food decreases in strength so that they need more and more of it to feel satisfied. Their studies show that in much the same way that people who abuse drugs and alcohol need increasingly large amounts over time, children who regularly eat ice cream also need more and more ice cream for their brains to indicate that they feel satisfied. This is unlikely to stop with ice cream.

Most of us can pinpoint a time of day, a particular day of the week or a mood when cravings kick in. These are often to do with lack of sleep, stress and strong emotions. The combination of fat and sugar seems to have a calming effect on the brain and carbohydrates boost our levels of serotonin, sometimes dubbed the 'happy hormone', so it is not surprising that we reach for the goodies when feeling out of sorts.

Chocolate is probably the most famous object of our desires and research has shown that it contains an estimated 380 chemicals. Some of them mimic the effects of our body's natural painkilling chemical opioids, other chemicals affect our levels of dopamine and yet others mimic the effects of cannabis. And we wonder why we like it so much!

I am not a fan of the ridiculous and completely impractical advice about how to reduce food cravings that are given in so many healthy eating and diet books. But even the brain scanning research seems to back up the advice that if you want to reduce food cravings you need to avoid your triggers.

Revenge of the Environment: Is Your Environment Killing You?

Research at the Monell Chemical Senses Centre suggests that our brains' memory centres are highly active during food cravings.[11] This would back up the notion that food cravings are more about the associations we make with a particular type of food: an emotion, a person, a time and/or a place. That could mean the drive home from work, that kick-off-the-shoes part of the evening, being in your childhood home, or simply standing near the goodies cupboard in your kitchen. Availability has a lot to answer for. Once your brain has had a little hit of dopamine from a salty or fatty snack in any one of these situations, it rapidly learns to link these bits of information – the place or time – and the good feelings. Knowing that those foods will be available to you again in that place or time puts enormous pressure on your reserves of willpower to work against your body's instinct to hoover up all things fatty and sugary in case of future famine. And, as we have seen, willpower is a limited commodity. Changing as much as you can of your environment to avoid as many of these temptations as possible is the first step towards lessening the burden on your willpower.

Do you really need twelve packs of crisps for the school lunches in your cupboard? They might be cheaper but just think how much misery they are causing you. If they have to stay can you leave them in your partner's car boot so they aren't as available to you?

If salty nibbles are your thing can you swap them for a lighter variety of crisps to be your Keepers?

Could you swap your latte for an Americano with plenty of hot milk in the coffee shop?

Many of these strategies might sound simplistic, but they address the main problem that several research studies have identified: seeing a trigger food makes it much more likely that a person will give in to the craving. Out of sight is now scientifically proven to be (more) out of mind. However, knowing that you have your Keeper(s) to look forward to should be enough to keep you away from temptation.

ATTENTION TO DETAIL

Making your environment more conducive to healthy eating is not just about *removing* temptation. Suggestions in the environment for eating the right stuff are so *incredibly* subtle it's hard to believe.

For me there is absolutely no point in buying those nets of oranges you get in the supermarket all year round even though they are usually cheap. I will never eat them. But just buying a few large juicy oranges that, most importantly, have that loose, easy peel skin, makes me crave them every time I'm looking for a snack. If they're not easy to peel I won't eat them. I also know that something as simple as having the fruit bowl bang in the centre of my counter top as opposed to somewhere even slightly more difficult to get to will foretell how much fruit I eat in a day.

It's the same with apples. Some varieties of apple could get the award for most boring fruit, while others are delicious. I've realised it is so well worth taking enough time to see which ones are in season and not just buying the ones that are marketed as being good for school lunch boxes or on special offer. If half of them rot at the bottom of the fruit bowl every week, don't waste your time on them.

Sticking cocktail sticks into a punnet of washed raspberries makes me far more likely to eat them, otherwise – even though I love them – I nearly always end up throwing some of them out after they have sat for too long in the fridge. I know that part of the reason is that, somewhere between the conscious and unconscious, I am put off by the chance of their juice staining my clothes. It just shows, the simplest changes have a huge effect on what I tuck into when the munchies strike!

So What Do We Do when a Craving Attacks?

One school of psychological thought would suggest that we put in place what is known as an 'Implementation Intention'. This is like a preconceived action plan for various situations we might encounter. These plans tend to take the form of 'If … then …' statements, so, for example, an individual might decide that if there is a bread basket on the table in a restaurant then they will ask for it to be removed so that they are not tempted. The idea behind this strategy is to take away the element of choice from some scenarios and to introduce a new automatic response. In the case of the bread basket this would help the person to avoid any internal mental chatter along the lines of 'Well, I haven't eaten much today … oh but I'm trying to cut down on carbs … yes but I'll probably order fish and vegetables so a little bread won't hurt … etc.'

Implementation intentions can reduce the mental stress involved in decision making and increase the overall weight loss.[12] But what is the best course of action to choose for your 'If … then …' action plan?

1   **Remove the temptation, or yourself:** As I have said, cravings attack most when something is available to us. If you know you have some tortilla chips left over from last night in the

cupboard or a fridge full of cheese, then these are likely to be calling you all day until you get rid of them. (I have a friend who pours washing-up liquid on top of any desserts she puts in the bin after having friends in to dinner to make sure they stay there. She says she had to do something when she noticed herself placing a dessert very gingerly in the bin and perfectly covered – just in case she changed her mind about throwing it out!) The other option is to remove yourself: get out of the room, perhaps telling yourself that if you still want them in half an hour you can have some. Chances are you will get distracted and your craving will pass.

2   **Have a little:** In a recent study carried out at the Cornell University Food and Brand Lab researchers discovered that food cravings can be satisfied with just a bite.[13] The researchers gave either small- or large-sized snacks to a group of 104 study participants. The people who ate the large snacks consumed seventy-seven per cent more calories than the small snack group, but after fifteen minutes both groups reported feeling the same levels of satiety and reduction in cravings. This and other studies show that if we just take a small bite, after fifteen minutes the cravings will be gone and we won't remember how much we ate or didn't eat.

3   **Substitute:** Taking a somewhat similar approach to the methadone treatment strategy for heroin abuse and choosing alternative foodstuffs that also give pleasure, like a water ice-type ice lolly instead of ice cream, is another way to beat cravings. Is a water ice-type lolly exactly what you desire? No, but it will tick the box of something sweet and refreshing to put into your mouth and do a lot less damage than the ice cream. You are unlikely to still crave the ice cream after you've had it. It's an enormous improvement and a lot more realistic than telling yourself you will swap the ice cream for a stick of celery. It is an exercise in damage limitation. It's also exactly what I talk about in the Fabulous Jelly programme – identifying your Keepers and finding *realistic* trade-offs. Your Keepers will act as a type of 'fair swap' for the many sugary and/ or fatty foods that you have been eating and will also be the carrot on a stick that you can look forward to in the very near future – as long as you don't indulge in dessert at the restaurant or half the sweet counter when you go to buy the newspaper. It's a *temporary* damage limitation exercise – in the future you will want to make even healthier choices.

4   **Postpone:** The idea of having some – but later is also supported by research.[14] The researchers asked participants in their study to imagine being offered a dessert from a restaurant-style dessert cart. They divided the participants into three groups: the first group were instructed to imagine choosing their favourite dessert and eating it, the second group were instructed to imagine that they had decided they would not eat dessert at all, and the third group were told to imagine that they had told themselves they would not have any now, but would later. Using questionnaires the researchers then measured how much the different groups were distracted by thoughts of food immediately afterwards. Normally any unfinished business tends to rattle around in our heads until we sort it out. It is what is known as the 'Zeigarnik effect' and most of us will have experienced it at least a few times in our lives – often when we are trying to sleep.[15] (If this does happen to you, write down what it is on your mind and that way the part of your brain that is working to keep this concern to the forefront of your mind, can rest easy.) According to this effect, the group who thought about having some dessert, but later, should have been most distracted by thoughts about having the food until the time that they actually ate it. Postponing the pleasure should have become the distracting thought. But it didn't. In fact, their results showed that it was less stressful for the brain to think 'I'll have some later' than 'I won't have any at all'. More surprisingly, when the researchers repeated this experiment using a bowl of M&Ms, the people who were instructed to tell themselves they would have some but later, did not over-indulge when the sneaky researchers later pretended the experiment was over and told them they could help themselves to the remaining M&Ms. Interestingly, the group who decided not to allow themselves to have any during the experiment helped themselves far more freely when the study was supposedly over.

Don't Give Up!

These results support the Fabulous Jelly recommendation not to give up anything. When it comes to eating, it is much less stressful for your brain to choose not to deny yourself some indulgences but instead to choose to have them 'later'.

Give up giving up. Don't try to 'give up' any food that you really like, but instead tell yourself that you can have a little of it sometimes – preferably not now.

Later, Rather Than Sooner – the Power of Will-power

In the 1960s an American psychologist by the

name of Walter Mischel of Stanford University ran experiments with young children to test the mental processes that allow some people to delay gratification.[16] A group of 653 four-year-old children were asked to choose something they liked from an assortment of biscuits, marshmallows and pretzels. They were then told by a researcher that he/she would leave them alone for an undisclosed period of time (which turned out to be fifteen minutes) and that if the child wanted to eat the chosen treat they could ring on a bell and the researcher would come back and allow them to indulge, but that if they could hold out until the researcher's return, they could choose a second treat from the tray. Of the 653 recruits, about thirty per cent managed to delay indulging, others didn't even wait to ring the bell, while the majority waited under three minutes before ringing the bell.

It wasn't until many years later that Mischel serendipitously noticed that these early results may prove to be indicators of later life events.[17] The children in the early studies were recruited from a school that Mischel's three daughters also attended. Over casual dinner conversation with his daughters, Mischel began to notice that the children who had been least able to delay eating their chosen sweet were having most difficulties in school in their teenage years. When the psychologist began to research this in more detail, using reports from parents and teachers and academic results, he found that the students who were least able to delay gratification experienced more behavioural problems in school and at home, lower academic scores, more difficulty maintaining friendships and struggled more with life stressors.

Now if you are mentally filing all of this information under the heading 'Not My Fault – Can't Do Anything About It', then stop right now. While it is true to say that the ability to put off eating until later is partially inherited, partially a result of your childhood and linked to a lower Body Mass Index (BMI) in adulthood, this doesn't give you a licence to blame genetics, parents and everyone but yourself. Remember what we are talking about here is essentially willpower and, like a muscle, it responds to exercise. Essentially you need to practise delaying eating in order to give yourself a feeling of being in control of, instead of controlled by, food. You could start by choosing to delay eating by five minutes, then six then seven and so on, or you can choose whatever time delays you wish.

The aim is simply to activate those areas of the

brain that we now know are involved in self-control, so that it becomes increasingly easy for the brain to fire that set of neurons associated with delayed gratification that simply makes you think 'waiting won't kill me'. You may, in fact, find that you get a bit of a kick out of a small delay that makes you feel in charge of your eating. It might be that that neural pathway in your brain is a 'road less travelled' and a bit of practice will make it a far easier ride for your brain to take in future.

When we were leaving school for the last time, one teacher gave some words of wisdom for those of us heading to college:

> *Ladies, love everyone in general, and no one in particular.*

Perhaps the same wisdom might apply to food!

11

FROM PAVLOV TO PAVLOVA

In the very early 1900s Ivan Pavlov, a Russian physio-
logist interested in digestion, discovered that a dog
could be taught ('conditioned') to salivate without any
sign of food.[18] In his lab a dog was placed in a sound-
proof, smell-proof cubicle. A sound was made when
food was given and the amount of saliva produced
by the dog was measured. After pairing the sound (a
bell) with the food a number of times, the researchers
then made the sound without giving the dog food
and the dog still salivated. This became known as
'Classical Conditioning'; the unconscious pairing of
two seemingly unrelated things, in this case a bell and
salivation. In fact, the dog continued to salivate many
times when the bell rang without food, until eventu-

ally he stopped. This was important research at the time because it showed that unconscious biological processes such as salivation can be conditioned to respond to external things unconsciously. This type of learning is the basis of how many phobias develop when a person unconsciously learns to associate an object such as a spider with fear, by observing the fear of a parent for example, or by listening to unhelpful stories about Little Miss Muffet from the age of two. It is, of course, also how we learn to feel suddenly hungry when we step into our mother's kitchen, or see an advertisement for a local bakery. We have been unconsciously conditioned.

But in a bit of a double whammy, not only can we be conditioned to feel what we think of as hunger through Classical Conditioning, we may also be taught to associate how to console ourselves with food. When a therapist wants to help a client to get rid of a phobia they might teach the person to relax in the presence of the trigger (such as a spider etc.) or teach them to associate the trigger with something more pleasant. In a similar vein, when your mother gave you that first biscuit because you were crying, frightened or hurt, you quickly learned to associate sweet treats with comfort and twenty years later you are still using the same self-comforting strategy.

Around the same time as Pavlov's famous work, Edward Thorndike was doing similar work on learning in the USA.[19] He showed that animals (and therefore presumably people) learn from the consequences of their behaviour. In what he called the 'Law of Effect', he said that any behaviour that is followed by positive consequences, or what he charmingly called 'a pleasant state of affairs', is likely to be repeated. This is hardly a huge surprise to us now, but it does explain why it is far easier for us to learn to use pleasurable food as a comfort when we are upset and also why we learn this association much faster than we learn good eating habits through repetition that doesn't feel like it is being rewarded.

Building on the principles of the Law of Effect, B. F. Skinner studied how rats could be trained (conditioned) to press a lever to get a reward (food pellet).[20] Although you may think that you have not quite lowered yourself to the level of food pellets, his research is really useful to understanding what's going on when diets go belly up.

Skinner found that:

1   Voluntary behaviour is reinforced by positive consequences and inhibited by negative consequences.

2   For a behaviour to be successfully reinforced the reward needs to be almost instantaneous.

3   Punishment makes a person try to avoid the punishment rather than stop the undesired behaviour.

In weight-loss terms this means that in order for healthy eating to be reinforced we need to get fast results so that we will keep going. It also means that every time we fall off the diet wagon we learn to hate diets (the punishment) rather than the unhealthy eating that caused our problem in the first place. Dieting, and the feelings of loss and failure that so often come with it, becomes what we want to avoid.

In order to reinforce our weight-loss efforts our minds need to see fast results. This way it will, first consciously and then unconsciously, pair 'new eating habits' with 'feel great', 'feel attractive', 'feel more agile', 'feel less breathless' and so on. For so long we have all been told about how weight loss needs to be slow and gradual in order to avoid slowing down our metabolism and if we lose weight too quickly we will only lose water, etc. It was a long time before I finally learned to do just what I knew was right for me and that was to get some weight off as fast as was healthily possible so that I had something worth protecting. It was only after my initial weight loss that I came across a study published in the highly prestigious *New England Journal of Medicine* to back up my theory.

Stop Press!

The study exploded a few weight-loss myths including the one that says that losing large amounts of weight quickly is always associated with poorer long-term weight loss than a more gradual weight loss. The authors concluded that sometimes a fad diet is just what you need to kick-start your weight loss. The authors also stated that you do not have to set moderate realistic weight-loss goals and that those who set extremely high goals and lose a lot of weight (some of which may be regained) are often still healthier/thinner than their counterparts who set more moderate weight-loss goals. The researchers concluded, however, that it probably varies for different people.[21]

The study debunks the assumption that all fast weight loss (I do not mean dangerously starving yourself) will result in eventual weight gain and frees us to look at it instead as a positive reinforcement for our efforts.

Some effort → Feel great → Continued effort

The Fabulous Jelly programme does not specify how much weight or what percentage of your body fat you should aim to lose or precisely how fast you should aim to lose it. That is up to you and you do have to use some common sense. Very extreme dieting is, of course, dangerous and will slow down your metabolism. What the programme does do is help you to work with your mind and unconscious instincts instead of against them.

IDENTIFYING YOUR KEEPERS AND CUTTING DOWN SIGNIFICANTLY ON CARBS WILL HELP YOU TO SEE WEIGHT LOSS AT A HEALTHY PACE AND GIVE YOU THE INCENTIVE YOU NEED TO KEEP GOING.

12

As Few Words as Possible on Stress

I don't want to repeat all the stuff you already know about stress being bad for you. But perhaps if you understand what is going on inside your body relating to weight loss and weight gain then you might be able to become aware of yourself when you reach for the salty, fatty or sugary snacks as stress hits.

Some Facts about Stress and Obesity

- Stress sets off our Fight or Flight response – in cavemen this was useful to give us an instant surge of energy to kill a lion or run like hell away from it.

- Acute, short-term stress can decrease appetite.

- Cortisol is the stress hormone that makes us look for high sugar or carbohydrate foods to replenish our energy stores when the stress is over or our energy stores (mental or physical) are depleted.

- To move the sugar ingested during these 'snack attacks' from our blood to the muscles we need insulin. High levels of insulin and sugar in the body increase fat storage.

- Cortisol can collect fat from the blood and other storage places and move it to the belly. It can also increase the size of fat cells.

- Abdominal fat, more than fat in any other part of the body, is linked to an increased risk of diabetes and heart disease.

- Unlike the caveman facing the lion, the stressful situations we encounter today don't give us an opportunity to work off the extra calories we consume: we don't tend to run around the kitchen, office or traffic jam to escape. Therefore the calories turn to fat.

- Sweet foods and fats have been shown to calm the stress response by increasing hormones related to positive moods.[22]

- Our brain is extremely clever: once it links the comfort of sugar or fat with a stressful situation it will trigger that response again even faster next time.

- A study showed that women are affected by more types of stress than men. In addition to financial and work stress, women tend to put on weight in response to family or relationship problems and hampered lifestyle circumstances. For men it showed that lack of decision-making authority and lack of interesting duties and opportunity to learn new skills resulted in weight gain.[23]

- However, although many studies have shown a link between stress and weight gain, a lot may be explained by behavioural factors (craving comfort food instead of relaxing with exercise). One study showed that only individuals who already had a raised BMI put on weight in response to stress.[24] Those with a low BMI actually decreased in weight. Stress causes not just a biological reason to put on weight but also increases the likelihood of fat-inducing behaviours such as craving high fat/sugar/salt foods.

- Lack of sleep affects our fat cells. Just four nights of only four-and-a-half hours sleep decreased the fat cell's responsiveness to insulin – the hormone that makes muscle, liver and fat cells take up glucose. If the glucose doesn't get absorbed and remains in the bloodstream the individual is at a higher risk of diabetes. Research linking lack of sleep with weight gain also suggests that leptin, the body's appetite-regulating hormone, is probably also negatively affected by lack of sleep.[25]

Becoming aware of what you are doing is the first step in making a conscious choice about whether or not you want to behave like a robot for the rest of your life, or perhaps choose to trade a very high fat content treat for a lesser evil. I know the diet books will tell you to reach instead for a piece of fruit or handful of nuts, but frankly I think you will be doing very well if you swap your 1,000-calorie helping of tortilla chips for two, or even three, bags of light crisps on your first attempt. Do this and you will avoid your trigger for all-or-nothing thinking. On your second attempt your brain will have remembered that feeling of a little bit of virtue without too much pain, with the result that next time you might actually manage to put the crisps in a bowl and sit down at a table to enjoy them. This way you might well manage to cut it down to just one or two packets of light crisps because you will probably eat them more slowly. On your next attempt you will have well and truly caught the bug for being able to allow yourself a wisely chosen treat and less of it, so that you get the reward or comfort without the quantity of calories. This is the Fabulous Jelly way of getting you jump-started. Choosing to look at even healthier ways from here on in is up to you.

Placing the crisps or alternative victim of your

voracious appetite in a bowl means that you are not having a quick and sneaky munch with your head in the treat cupboard so that others don't see you.

IN NO DIET OR BIOLOGY BOOK DOES IT STATE THAT CALORIES CONSUMED WITHOUT BEING SEEN = NO WEIGHT GAIN. THIS SEEMS TO BE A WELL KEPT SECRET OF THE DIETING COMMUNITY ALONE.

We all behave ourselves better when we know we are being watched. We actually twig this one in early childhood and it's downhill from there. Put masks on people and you can completely change how they conduct themselves in a very short space of time. A hoodie pulled up over a teenage boy's (or anyone's) head has the same effect of making them feel anonymous, freer and less tied by the guiding morals and ethics they normally live their lives by. In fact, we even behave better in front of a mirror as the mirror forces us to look at ourselves, which is very uncomfortable if we are doing something we are ashamed of – like pigging out. Go ahead and experiment with this yourself. Studies have shown that a person will make fewer illicit visits to the fridge when they have placed a mirror on the door. Or you could try placing a stand-up mirror on the table facing where you sit so that you can see yourself eating. This is a great way of making you aware of your eating and to introduce a bit of mindfulness to your mealtime, which, by no coincidence, is what I want to talk about next.

13

INSTRUCTIONS ON HOW TO WAKE A SLEEPING PILOT

One of the cornerstones of cognitive behavioural therapy is realising that thoughts are not facts, they are just thoughts. This is a revelation for many people who had never looked at their mental rumblings in this way and it often gives the person a sudden feeling of freedom when they realise that their thoughts are, in fact, just one way of looking at things. Mindfulness is a type of meditation that also emphasises this separation from our not always impressive mental machinations. Mindfulness has its roots in Buddhism (although similar approaches are also seen in Christian meditations), but is now taught as a secular exercise. The practice teaches the individual to observe the constant stream of thoughts that pass through their mind without becoming involved with them. It's a bit like learning to watch thoughts come and go as if they were ships passing, without jumping on board. This practice helps to separate the mind from the body and aims to get the person 're-attached' to their body, instead of living in their heads as most of us do in our busy lives. So what does this have to do with eating?

You are probably a lot more aware of what *mindlessness* is: those times when you do something that perhaps you have done a thousand times before, and which you now carry out while mentally 'on auto-pilot'. Like eating. All you really need to do is shovel food from the plate to your mouth, which leaves your mind free to channel surf, read or attempt one-handed typing. The problem with this is, of course, that we pay no attention to the flavours in the food, or when we have had enough. Eating mindfully means becoming aware of every sensation that you experience through your five senses, both internally and externally. Eating too quickly is one of the big offenders when it comes to weight gain as it nearly always causes us to overeat. Mindfulness not only slows us down when eating but also adds a feeling of actually savouring and enjoying the whole experience rather than just refuelling.

When was the last time you considered your mid-week dinner to be an 'experience'? The distinction is something similar to the difference between a dull Tuesday evening dinner at home (most people hate Tuesdays most) versus getting on the glad rags and going to dinner in a restaurant you have never eaten in before. In the latter case you are more aware of what you are wearing, the decor, the table setting, the staff, the lighting, the menu etc. You naturally become much more aware of each moment as the evening evolves than when you are at home. It's not that you need to go through every moment of your day mind-fully, but doesn't it sound tempting to think that every night when you get into bed you could pinpoint say, five moments during that day that you were really attentive to and appreciative of?

If you have ever wondered where all the years have gone or felt that you daydream your life away going over the past or worrying about the future, then mindfulness will help. Because this form of meditation teaches the person to become alert to the present moment (it is not relaxation but can feel very pleasant), they stop losing each moment by worrying or planning other moments that have either passed or not happened yet. To me this aspect in itself makes it well worth doing. Imagine being able to look back in the future and feel that you really lived, appreciated and enjoyed every second with your children, of your career or time with a loved one.

It does take a while to remember to practise mindfulness during your daily life, even if at the start you only practise it while brushing your teeth. But there is no grading of a good meditation or a bad one; the only difference between an experienced meditator and a novice is that the former will have learned to accept and not try to change the constant intrusion of thoughts that pass through their mind. The novice will tend to jump on board and get carried away with a thought and then get annoyed with themselves for doing so. Experience teaches you to be more accepting of this tendency.

The best way to learn mindfulness is by doing an eight-week mindfulness course which normally involves one two-hour session each week plus daily home practice. You can look online for a course near you (or check out www.fabulousjelly.ie for information on courses I will be running). I would also recommend that you read Jon Kabat Zinn's *Full Catastrophe Living* to really understand the benefits of mindfulness before embarking on any course.[26]

GRADUAL CHANGES WORK

I can't believe that I can go in and out of the kitchen 100 times a day without having the slightest temptation to snack on something. I get such a kick out of that.

I haven't eaten a bar of chocolate in months either, yet I never said I would give it up. I haven't given it up. I will sometimes have one or two chocolates when given a present of a box and the odd after dinner chocolate. But these things were never a problem anyway. It was the whole 'buying myself a bar of chocolate when I was on my own thing'. The 'me time' was a huge part of my 'having a bar' experience/routine. It was a symbol of downtime – even if that downtime was only three minutes.

I know I wouldn't have been able to do this without my Keepers. They have worked incredibly well for me. They don't have the same addictive quality to me but are something I can enjoy as a treat. Life isn't supposed to be boot camp so I don't feel in the least bit guilty about these.

> Am I ever tempted to buy a bar of chocolate? I really can't believe I'm saying this but no, not so far. But I will sometime and I will probably be a bit nervous of it. I now know it really does have an addictive quality to it that sets my brain bouncing off the inner walls of my head.

Having come to this stage in the book, you will have already moved yourself along the (re-)learning process of learning that can be divided into four stages:[27]

1 Unconscious Incompetence – this is when you don't even know that you don't know. For example, until you read this book you may not know just how many mental processes affect your ability to stick to an eating plan. Up until the first time you thought to yourself 'stuff this, it's too hard' during your first attempt to lose weight, you may have thought it was a simple matter of a once-off diet.

2 Conscious Incompetence – This is when you know you don't know. You have fallen off the wagon a few times or have had limited success and are now looking for an understanding of why.

3 Conscious Competence – this is probably where you are now or will be as soon as you take a few gentle steps on the Fabulous Jelly programme. You have gained an understanding of why you struggle with your weight but it will still take conscious effort to put into practice all of the things you have learned.

4 Unconscious Competence – the Holy Grail of eating, this is when you can control your eating naturally without any conscious effort – or it may be more realistic to say, with only as much conscious effort as any naturally good eater puts into choosing the right foods for themselves. Keep going – you'll get there!

14

SO THERE YOU HAVE IT AND HERE YOU ARE

So, now you have read the Fabulous Jelly programme. What's next for you? I hope that you have a feeling that you can start making a difference *right now* – no need to wait until tomorrow. I have covered a lot of material in this book and it is unlikely that you will remember it all without a few re-reads.

My aim in writing this book is to offer those who struggle with their weight an understanding of the multitude of biological and psychological factors that they need to factor in when trying to lose weight. Most healthy eating programmes and diet books only give the ideal eating plan without any reference to what's realistically possible for most of us. Because of this there has been what I see as a big motivational gap between what we know we should be eating and what we do eat. If nothing else I want the reader to come away from this book with an appreciation of just how much they were trying to swim against the tide in previous diets by paying absolutely no attention to their unconscious instincts and habits of thinking. I hope that after reading *Fabulous Jelly*, you will have an appreciation of the phenomenal complexity and what I consider the fascinating beauty of your brain and, most of all, a bit of kindness towards yourself for what you have put yourself through mentally and physically on previous diets. You're a saint to be still reading anything on the subject of weight loss!

The premise of the Fabulous Jelly programme is simple: work with, not against, your unconscious mind. You really have no choice. It controls everything you do, think and feel. Obviously then, you need to know what it's about and what it needs. You need to know that it considers change and weight loss to be a threat to your safety and existence and therefore isn't a big fan.

You need to know that all of your thoughts, beliefs and opinions are just one way of viewing the world – they are not facts. If they are not getting you where you want to go you need to change them. They were probably someone else's to begin with.

You need to know that you are not weak because your willpower fails you sometimes. It happens to everyone and, therefore, you should not rely on willpower alone to form the basis of any new eating plan. Such a plan will fail. Instead you need to gently guide your unconscious mind to seeing the benefits of small changes in your eating habits in the form of relatively fast weight loss and the boost to energy and self-esteem that comes with it. These are things that appeal to the unconscious as they are also relevant to your survival. It becomes a fair trade-off.

You need to accept that your life is your life at the moment and you need to work with what you have while losing weight. It is pointless to take on eating plans that demand time that you don't have, energy that you don't have or, indeed, money that you don't have. However, with weight loss comes increased confidence, energy and social interaction. Life can change simply because you have lost weight.

The Fabulous Jelly programme aims to give you the motivation to start losing weight without any all-or-nothing thinking about being 'on' or 'off' a diet. You can use the programme to get you within the guideline range of weight for your age and height (BMI) or just to kick-start your healthy eating plan before you join a weight-loss club or embark on a more specific eating plan. It is not about getting you a beach body. Neither do I pretend that the way you eat on the programme is a medium- or long-term eating plan. It is simply a negotiation – a mid-way point between what you are eating now and what you should be eating. I found that once I had lost some weight I naturally looked to increasingly healthy foods.

Now it's your turn to get going on giving yourself some weight loss a.s.a.p.

Don't forget to:

1 Identify your Keepers

2 Swap and tweak – and most of all reduce your carbs

3 Keep a food diary

4 Get some exercise

With practice, you will learn to notice your habits in thinking and to differentiate between those that are useful and those that have never served you well. You will enjoy the sense of being a manager rather than a victim of *your choice* to lose weight. And you will enjoy the feeling of being able to live your life to the full while staying within the Fabulous Jelly guidelines.

Most of all, I hope that you find that the Fabulous Jelly programme rids you of any guilt or sense of failure for previous failed attempts at weight loss. I hope now you understand that this was the fault of those programmes, not of you.

This is your time. Go Do It!

God bless,

Susannah

REFERENCES

1   www.facts.randomhistory.com/human-brain-facts.html.

2   This is an example of a Cognitive Behavioural Therapy approach. For more see William T. O'Donoghue & Jane E. Fisher, *Cognitive Behaviour Therapy* (2008, Wiley and Sons Inc., New Jersey).

3   www.blogs.ucl.ac.uk/hbrc/2012/06/29/busting-the-21-days-habit-formation-myth/.

4   Gerry Duffy, *Who Dares, Runs* (2011, Ballpoint Press, Bray).

5   Amy Chua, *Battle Hymn of the Tiger Mother* (2011, Penguin, New York).

6   Roy F. Baumeister & John Tierney, *Willpower. Rediscovering the Greatest Human Strength* (2011, Penguin, London).

7   William M. Hedgcock, Kathleen D. Vohs & Akshay R. Rao, 'Reducing self-control depletion effects through enhanced sensitivity to implementation: Evidence from fMRI and behavioral studies', *Journal of Consumer Psychology* 22(4), 2012, pp. 486–95.

8   Kathleen D. Vohs, Roy F. Baumeister, N. L. Mead, S. Ramanathan & B. J. Schmeichel, 'Engaging in Self-Control Heightens Urges and Feelings'. Cited in Roy F. Baumeister & John Tierney, *Willpower. Why Self Control is the Secret to Success* (2012, Penguin, London).

9   Susan Yanovski, 'Sugar and Fat: Cravings and Aversions',
    The Journal of Nutrition 133(3), March 2003 (accessible at
    http://jn.nutrition.org/cgi/content/full/133/3/835S).

10 G. J. Wang, N. D. Volkow, F. Telang, M. Jayne & M. Rao,
    2003, 'Exposure to Appetitive Food Stimuli Markedly
    Activates the Human Brain', *NeuroImage* 21(4), 2004, pp.
    1790–97.

11 Marcia Levin Pelchat, Andrea Johnson, Robin Chan,
    Jeffrey Valdez & J. Daniel Ragland, 'Images of Desire:
    Food Craving Activation During fMRI', *NeuroImage* 23,
    2004, pp. 1486–93.

12 Aleksandra Luszczynska, Anna Sobczyk & Charles
    Abraham, 'Planning to Lose Weight: Randomized
    Controlled Trial of an Implementation Intention Prompt
    to Enhance Weight Reduction among Overweight and
    Obese Women', *Health Psychology* (26)4, July 2007, pp.
    507–12.

13 Ellen Van Kleef, Sjimizu Mitsusra & Brian Wansink,
    'Just a Bite: Considerably Smaller Snack Portions
    Satisfy Delayed Hunger and Cravings', *Food Quality and
    Preference*, 27(1), 2013, pp. 96–100.

14 Nicole L. Mead & Vanessa M. Patrick, 'In Praise of
    Putting Things Off: Postponing Consumption Pleasures
    Facilitates Self-Control', 22 June 2012 (abstract available
    at http://ssrn.com/abstract=2089152). Cited in Roy F.
    Baumeister & John Tierney, *Willpower. Why Self Control
    is the Secret to Success* (2012, Penguin, London).

15   The effect is named after Bluma Zeigarnik (1900–88), who first identified the effect in her 1927 doctoral thesis.

16   Walter Mischel & Ozlem Ayduk, 'Willpower in a Cognitive-Affective Processing System: The Dynamics of Delay of Gratification', in Roy F. Baumeister & Kathleen Vohs (eds), *Handbook of Self Regulation: Research, Theory and Applications* (2004, Guilford, New York). Cited in Roy F. Baumeister & John Tierney, *Willpower. Why Self Control is the Secret to Success* (2012, Penguin, London).

17   Yuichi Shoda, Walter Mischel & Philip K. Peake, 'Predicting Adolescent Cognitive and Self-Regulatory Competencies from Preschool Delay of Gratification: Identifying Diagnostic Conditions', *Developmental Psychology* 26, 1990, pp. 978–86.

18   Ivan Petrovich Pavlov, *Conditional Reflexes*, edited and translated by G. V. Anrep (1927, Oxford University Press, Oxford).

19   Edward Lee Thorndike, *Animal Intelligence: Experimental Studies* (1911, Macmillan, New York).

20   B. F. Skinner, *The Behavior of Organisms: An Experimental Analysis* (1938, Appleton-Century, New York).

21   K. Casazza *et al.*, 'Myths, Presumptions and Facts about Obesity', *New England Journal of Medicine*, 368(5), 2013, pp. 446–54.

22   R. J. Wurtman, J. J. Wurtman, M. M. Regan, J. M. McDermott, R. H. Tsay & J. J. Breu, 'Effects of Normal Meals Rich in Carbohydrates or Proteins on Plasma

Tryptophan and Tyrosine Ratios', *American Journal of Clinical Nutrition* 77, 2003, pp. 128–32.

23 Jason P. Block, Yulei He, Alan M. Zaslavsky, Lin Ding & John Z. Ayanian, 'Psychosocial Stress and Change in Weight among US Adults', *American Journal of Epidemiology* 170(2), 2009, pp. 181–92.

24 M. Kivimaki, J. Head, J. E. Ferrie, M. J. Shipley, E. Brunner, J. Vahtera & M. G. Marmot, 'Work Stress, Weight Gain and Weight Loss: Evidence for Bidirectional Effects of Job Stress on Body Mass Index in the Whitehall II Study', *International Journal of Obesity* 30, 2006, pp. 982–7.

25 S. Taheri, L. Lin, D. Austin, T. Young & E. Mignot, 'Short Sleep Duration is Associated with Reduced Leptin, Elevated Ghrelin, and Increased Body Mass Index' (accessible at: www.plosmedicine.org/article/info:doi/10.1371/journal.pmed.0010062).

26 Jon Kabat-Zinn, *Full Catastrophe Living: How to Cope with Stress, Pain and Illness Using Mindfulness Meditation* (2001, Piaktus, London).

27 Noel Burch, 'The Four Stages for Learning Any New Skill', http://www.gordontraining.com/free-workplace-articles/learning-a-new-skill-is-easier-said-than-done/.

ACKNOWLEDGEMENTS

I want to thank all the team at Mercier Press for giving me the opportunity to commit to paper all the ideas which rattled around my head for so long, so that they may now rattle around your head for the foreseeable future. My thanks to Mary Feehan for the good humour and the instant welcome that she bestowed upon me. Thanks to Niamh Hatton who lent her expertise to my initial manuscript and helped it to take shape. Also, to Wendy Logue who continued the process, showing endless patience with this first-time author. I am grateful to Rachel Hutchings whose attention to grammatical detail I really enjoyed even when it slightly hurt my pride. I wish the reader could have seen all of the creative and artistic ideas that came from the fabulous jelly of Sarah O'Flaherty who designed the cover – thanks Sarah. Also, my thanks to Patrick Dunphy for his high energy and knowledge in the marketing sphere and to Sharon O'Donovan who took *Fabulous Jelly* to far-flung booksellers. My thanks to all the Mercier Press team for making the writing of this book such a great experience.

I want to thank my husband Arthur Ryan, not only for allowing me to almost disappear for several weeks so that I could concentrate on writing, but also for being my best friend. Arthur makes even Tuesdays fun (Tuesdays are semi-scientifically proven to be the most boring day of the week). To my boys Arthur, Oliver and Chester, you make me so proud. I love you all madly.

It is impossible to properly express my gratitude to my darling parents for everything you have done for me and everything you have given me – most of all your constant love. All I can do is to say publicly here how much I love you both.